DATE DUE

HIGHSMITH 45-220

LESBIAN HEALTH

Current Assessment and Directions for the Future

Andrea L. Solarz, *Editor*

Committee on Lesbian Health Research Priorities

Neuroscience and Behavioral Health Program

Health Sciences Policy Program

Health Sciences Section

INSTITUTE OF MEDICINE

NATIONAL ACADEMY PRESS
Washington, D.C. 1999

National Academy Press • 2101 Constitution Avenue, N.W. • Washington, DC 20418

NOTICE: The project that is the subject of this report was approved by the Governing Board of the National Research Council, whose members are drawn from the councils of the National Academy of Sciences, the National Academy of Engineering, and the Institute of Medicine. The members of the committee responsible for the report were chosen for their special competences and with regard for appropriate balance.

The Institute of Medicine was chartered in 1970 by the National Academy of Sciences to enlist distinguished members of the appropriate professions in the examination of policy matters pertaining to the health of the public. In this, the Institute acts under both the Academy's 1863 congressional charter responsibility to be an adviser to the federal government and its own initiative in identifying issues of medical care, research, and education. Dr. Kenneth I. Shine is president of the Institute of Medicine.

This study was supported by Task Order No. 27, under Contract No. N01-OD-4-2139 from the Office of Research on Women's Health at the National Institutes of Health.

Library of Congress Cataloging-in-Publication Data

Lesbian health : current assessment and directions for the future /
Andrea L. Solarz, editor ; Committee on Lesbian Health Research
Priorities, Neuroscience and Behavioral Health Program [and] Health
Sciences Policy Program, Health Sciences Section, Institute of
Medicine.
    p. cm.
    Report based on a workshop held in Oct. 1997.
    Includes bibliographical references (p.   ) and index.
    ISBN 0-309-06093-1 (case)
    ISBN 0-309-06567-4 (perfect)
    1. Lesbians—Health and hygiene. 2. Lesbians—Health and
hygiene—Government policy—United States. I. Solarz, Andrea L. II.
Institute of Medicine (U.S.). Committee on Lesbian Health Research
Priorities.
    RA564.87 .L46 1999
    613'.086'643—dc21   99-6101

Additional copies of this report are available for sale from the National Academy Press, 2101 Constitution Avenue, N.W., Lock Box 285, Washington, DC 20055. Call (800) 624-6242 or (202) 334-3313 (in the Washington metropolitan area), or visit the NAP on-line bookstore at **www.nap.edu.**

For more information about the Institute of Medicine, visit the IOM home page at **www2.nas.edu/iom.**

Printed in the United States of America

The serpent has been a symbol of long life, healing, and knowledge among almost all cultures and religions since the beginning of recorded history. The image adopted as a logotype by the Institute of Medicine is based on a relief carving from ancient Greece, now held by the Staatliche Museen in Berlin.

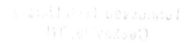

COMMITTEE ON LESBIAN HEALTH RESEARCH PRIORITIES

ANN W. BURGESS (*Chair*), Professor, University of Pennsylvania School of Nursing
JUDITH BRADFORD,★ Director, Survey and Evaluation Research Laboratory, Virginia Commonwealth University
DONNA JEAN BROGAN, Professor, Biostatistics Department, Rollins School of Public Health, Emory University
SAMUEL R. FRIEDMAN, Senior Research Fellow, National Development and Research Institutes, Inc., New York
CYNTHIA A. GÓMEZ, Assistant Adjunct Professor, Center for AIDS Prevention Studies, University of California at San Francisco
IRIS F. LITT, Professor of Pediatrics and Director, Division of Adolescent Medicine, Stanford University School of Medicine
BRUCE S. McEWEN, Professor and Laboratory Head, Laboratory of Endocrinology, Rockefeller University
LARRY NORTON, Chief, Breast Cancer Medicine, Memorial Sloan-Kettering Cancer Center, New York
GLORIA E. SARTO, Professor, Department of Obstetrics and Gynecology, University of Wisconsin Hospital, Madison

Institute of Medicine Study Staff
ANDREA L. SOLARZ, Study Director (until July 1998)
CARRIE E. INGALLS, Research Associate (until August 1997)
THOMAS J. WETTERHAN, Research Assistant (until September 1998)
AMELIA B. MATHIS, Project Assistant
CHERYL MITCHELL, Administrative Assistant (until June 1998)
CONSTANCE M. PECHURA, Director, Neuroscience and Behavioral Health Program (until May 1998)

Copy Editor
FLORENCE POILLON

Health Sciences Section Staff
CHARLES H. EVANS, Jr., Head, Health Sciences Section
LINDA DEPUGH, Administrative Assistant
CARLOS GABRIEL, Financial Associate
ANDREW POPE, Director, Health Sciences Policy Program
VALERIE SETLOW, Director, Division of Health Sciences Policy (until October 1997)

★Resigned December 10, 1998.

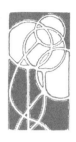

Reviewers

This report has been reviewed in draft form by individuals chosen for their diverse perspectives and technical expertise, in accordance with procedures approved by the National Research Council's Report Review Committee. The purpose of this independent review is to provide candid and critical comments that will assist the Institute of Medicine in making the published report as sound as possible and to ensure that the report meets institutional standards for objectivity, evidence, and responsiveness to the study charge. The review comments and draft manuscript remain confidential to protect the integrity of the deliberative process. The committee wishes to thank the following individuals for their participation in the review of this report:

GEORGE J. ANNAS, Boston University School of Public Health
RONALD W. ESTABROOK, University of Texas Southwestern
  Medical Center at Dallas
JOHN FLETCHER, University of Virginia (retired)
LUELLA KLEIN, Emory University School of Medicine
ED LAUMANN, University of Chicago
VICKIE MAYS, University of California, Los Angeles
HENRY W. RIECKEN, University of Pennsylvania

JEROME STRAUSS, University of Pennsylvania Medical Center
JOYCELYN WHITE, Legacy Good Samaritan Hospital

While the individuals listed above have provided constructive comments and suggestions, it must be emphasized that responsibility for the final content of this report rests entirely with the authoring committee and the Institute of Medicine.

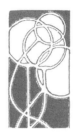

Preface

Women's health is a relatively new focus of research study. Theories about human health in general have traditionally been developed from studies of men. In recent years, research has expanded to include an explicit focus on women's health, as well as the inclusion of women in gender-neutral studies to ensure that findings may be applied broadly and appropriately. During the past two decades the unique health needs of a subgroup of women—lesbians—have been identified for study. Until this time, avoidance and silence dominated both professional and societal attitudes toward lesbian health needs.

Lesbians are found among all subpopulations of women. Lesbians are as diverse as the general population of all women, and they are represented in all racial and ethnic groups, all socioeconomic strata, and all ages. There is no single type of family, community, culture, or demographic category characteristic of lesbian women.

Research about lesbians has been conducted in a systematic fashion only since the 1950s. Tully (1995) has traced the historical development of the lesbian research literature over the past four decades. Initially, research focused on "lesbian etiology," or the factors that would cause a woman to be a lesbian. The next major phase of research, from the 1960s to the 1980s, explored psychological functioning of lesbians, typically by comparing nonclinical samples of lesbian and heterosexual women to determine whether being lesbian was a form of psychopathology. During the 1970s, researchers—who were often lesbians themselves—began to focus on lesbians as psychologically healthy individuals and to study their social functioning. Research since the 1980s has begun to examine issues related to the development of lesbians across their life spans.

Until the 1980s, few health care professionals discussed the similarities or differences between lesbians and other women. It was not until 1985 that a high level of interest in lesbian health emerged coincident with the design and implementation of the National Lesbian Health Care Survey (Bradford and Ryan, 1988). This survey provided a systematic approach to identify the health needs and concerns of lesbians. It also sought to underline the importance of studying lesbians and their health needs in order to improve health care delivery to them. Since then, other scholars and researchers have focused their efforts on this aspect of women's health. As a result, a body of knowledge has begun to develop.

Although there had been efforts to address issues specific to lesbian health over the past several decades, federal action was limited. In 1993, a meeting was held between representatives of national and local lesbian and gay health organizations and Secretary of Health and Human Services Donna Shalala, during which lesbian health activists asked that the Department of Health and Human Services (DHHS) increase its attention to, and better meet the health needs of, lesbians, gay men, bisexuals, and transgender individuals (Plumb, 1997). Subsequently, in February 1994 a Lesbian Health Roundtable, involving more than 60 lesbian and bisexual women's health activists from around the country, was held in Washington, D.C., to formalize the recommendations to DHHS and to establish a lesbian health agenda. The agenda subsequently presented to DHHS had as a priority the expansion of research on lesbian health issues.

Several federal initiatives emerged out of these meetings. In 1994, supplemental financing was provided for researchers funded by the National Institutes of Health (NIH) to support the inclusion of lesbian and bisexual women in ongoing studies, and questions about sexual behavior were added to the NIH Women's Health Initiative (WHI), a large longitudinal study and randomized clinical trial of women's health. Also as a result of these meetings, the NIH Office of Research on Women's Health requested that the Institute of Medicine (IOM) conduct a workshop to examine the need for future research on the health of lesbians, focusing on existing data and evaluating research methodologies. This workshop study is the result of that request.

Each section of this report presents ideas and perspectives the committee hopes will energize health professionals, researchers, policy makers, and others interested in lesbian health to face the challenges and opportunities of the new millennium.

Acknowledgments: This report reflects the dedication and thoughtfulness of a great many people. Each member of the Committee on Lesbian Health Research Priorities contributed to the deliberations by leading discussions, providing background references, and reading and commenting on report drafts. However, many other people also contributed to the project in numerous ways. The committee especially thanks the workshop participants for sharing their expertise—our work was enhanced by their presentations and their comments (see Appendixes B and C for the workshop agenda and participants, respectively). The committee heard testimony at the workshop and received written comments from a number of individuals and organizations (see Appendixes A and D for a selected bibliography and a list of those who provided testimony, respectively). This information was extremely useful in expanding our understanding of the issues and of the concerns of the lesbian health community. Numerous people also contributed background materials to the committee. We are especially grateful to Marjorie Plumb, formerly with the National Gay and Lesbian Medical Association, and Suzanne Haynes, now with the DHHS Office of Women's Health, for the materials they made available, and to Devi O'Neill for the notebook full of medical literature on lesbian health that she gave to the committee. Janine Cogan and Clinton Anderson of the American Psychological Association and Tracey St. Pierre of the Human Rights Campaign were also quite helpful in providing resources and information. Several individuals—often on short notice—were especially helpful in sharing their unpublished research or other background materials with the committee, including Deborah Bybee, Charlotte Patterson, and Deborah Bowen. The committee also appreciates the help that Marj Plumb provided as liaison to the lesbian community. In addition, we are grateful to Julie Honnold at the Survey and Evaluation Research Laboratory (SERL) and the Department of Sociology and Anthropology at Virginia Commonwealth University for her work on developing the sexual orientation cube data presented in Chapter 1, as well as to Arnold Overby, the computer network administrator at SERL, for his help with this task.

The committee is indebted to the IOM staff who worked on the project: Study Director Andrea Solarz, for her patience and skill in translating the workshop proceedings and committee discussions into a report; Constance Pechura who, during her tenure as director of the Division of Neuroscience and Behavioral Health, shared her broad understanding of the committee process with us; Research Assistant Thomas Wetterhan, who provided invaluable help in locating background materials, checking references, and preparing the draft document for publication; Project Assistant Amelia Mathis, for her hard work in setting up meetings, arranging travel and lodging, and preparing agenda materials; and Research Associate Carrie Ingalls who was especially helpful at the initial stages of the project in locating background materials.

Finally, the committee is grateful for the support and encouragement of the sponsors of the workshop study and for the interest of Vivian Pinn, Director of the NIH Office of Research on Women's Health, and of program officers Joyce Rudick, also from the Office of Research on Women's Health, and Wanda Jones, formerly associate director for Women's Health at the Centers for Disease Control and Prevention and now Deputy Assistant Secretary for Women's Health, DHHS.

Ann Burgess, D.N.Sc.
Chair

REFERENCES

Bradford J, and Ryan C. 1988. *The National Lesbian Health Care Survey: Final Report.* Washington, DC: National Lesbian and Gay Health Foundation.

Plumb M. 1997. Statement of the Gay and Lesbian Medical Association to the IOM Committee on Lesbian Health Research Priorities Regarding Community Perspective, Washington, DC.

Tully CT. 1995. In sickness and in health: Forty years of research on lesbians. In: Tully CT, ed. *Lesbian Social Services: Research Issues.* New York: Harrington Park Press/ Haworth Press, Inc. Pp. 1–18.

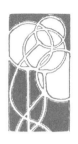

Contents

TABLES, FIGURES, AND BOXES

Tables

Contents

Figures

Boxes

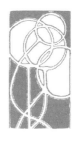

Acronyms

AIDS	Acquired immune deficiency syndrome
audio-CASI	Audio computer-assisted self-interview
BMI	Body mass index
BV	Bacterial vaginosis
CARDIA	Coronary Artery Risk Development in Young Adults
CDC	Centers for Disease Control and Prevention
DHHS	Department of Health and Human Services
FBI	Federal Bureau of Investigation
HIV	Human immunodeficiency virus
HPV	Human papillomavirus
ICD	International Classification of Diseases
IDU	Injection drug user
IOM	Institute of Medicine
MLHS	Michigan Lesbian Health Survey

NHANES	National Health and Nutrition Examination Survey
NHIS	National Health Interview Survey
NHS-II	Nurses' Health Study II
NHSDA	National Household Survey on Drug Abuse
NHSLS	National Health and Social Life Survey
NIAID	National Institute of Allergy and Infectious Diseases
NICHD	National Institute of Child Health and Human Development
NIDA	National Institute on Drug Abuse
NIH	National Institutes of Health
NIMH	National Institute of Mental Health
NLHCS	National Lesbian Health Care Survey
NORC	National Opinion Research Center
SAMHSA	Substance Abuse and Mental Health Services Administration
SERL	Survey and Evaluation Research Laboratory
SES	Socioeconomic status
STD	Sexually transmitted disease
T-ACASI	Telephone audio computer-assisted self-interview
WHI	Women's Health Initiative
WSW	Women who have sex with women
YWCA	Young Women's Christian Association

LESBIAN
HEALTH

Current Assessment and
Directions for the Future

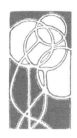

Executive Summary

Despite growing attention to research on women's health over the past decade, the health problems of some subgroups of women have continued to receive relatively little attention. Lesbians are one such subgroup. Although the body of research on lesbian health is growing, much of the research to date has methodological limitations, such as the lack of appropriate comparison groups, that make it difficult to draw clear conclusions about the health status and health risks of this group of women.

The Institute of Medicine (IOM) Committee on Lesbian Health Research Priorities was convened in July 1997 to:

1. assess the strength of the science base regarding the physical and mental health of lesbians,
2. review the methodological challenges involved in conducting research on lesbian health, and
3. suggest areas for research attention.

The study was funded by the National Institutes of Health (NIH) Office of Research on Women's Health, with the Centers for Disease Control and Prevention (CDC) also contributing funding through the NIH.

A primary charge of the committee was to organize and convene an invitational workshop to examine these issues. The workshop, held in October 1997, focused on the challenges involved in designing and conducting research on lesbian health, some of the contextual issues that can make it more difficult to conduct such research, and lesbians' risk for particular health conditions including cancer, mental health problems, substance abuse, HIV infection, and sexually transmitted diseases. Lesbians' use of and access to health care services were also discussed. The workshop involved 21 invited speakers, public testimony from more than a dozen presenters, and approximately 50 interested members of the public who also participated in the discussion.

This report is based on the committee's deliberations and reflects its review and evaluation of the scientific literature on lesbian health and of information presented at the workshop. The committee's conclusions and recommendations, which are outlined here, are presented in detail in the full report. It is important to recognize that this is a workshop-study report with recommendations and that the committee's information gathering and deliberations were thus limited compared to those of a full IOM study.

The committee identified several important reasons for directing attention to the study of lesbian health issues:

- **To gain knowledge to improve the health status and health care of lesbians.** Lesbians share many health risks and experiences in the health care system with women in general. For lesbians' health care to be both cost-effective and appropriate, the scope of their health problems must be better understood. Knowledge of areas in which the health of lesbians differs from that of other women may provide insights to improve the health of all women.

- **To confirm beliefs and to counter misconceptions about the health risks of lesbians.** In the face of little empirical information, there are numerous beliefs, myths, and misconceptions about the health risks of lesbians that can affect their health outcomes. These beliefs are often shared both by health care providers and by lesbians themselves. Some of these beliefs may be true; others are not. These beliefs include perceptions that lesbians do not need regular Pap tests or routine gynecological care, that they do not contract HIV/AIDS, and that there is an epidemic of breast cancer in the lesbian community.

• **To identify health conditions for which lesbians are at risk or tend to be at greater risk than heterosexual women or women in general.** A large body of epidemiological research has identified factors that place people at risk for health and mental health problems, with gender differences existing for many of these risk factors. However, because information about subjects' sexual preferences has not been collected in these studies, it is not possible to determine whether the lesbians who presumably are included in the samples differed from or were like other women with respect to these risk factors. In fact, some factors assumed to place women at risk for or to protect them against health disorders might not be present at the same levels or operate in the same ways for lesbians. In addition to facing many of the same stressors as heterosexual women, women who self-identify as lesbian may also experience stressors not commonly faced by heterosexual women, such as "stigmatization" both within and outside the health care setting. It is important to identify and understand those factors that are unique to lesbians and their impact on health.

The committee spent a significant amount of time discussing how to define lesbian sexual orientation. There is no standard definition of what constitutes a "lesbian." In general, sexual orientation is most often described as including behavioral, affective (i.e., desire or attraction), and cognitive (i.e., identity) dimensions that occur along continua (Laumann et al., 1994). Women may exhibit differing degrees of same-sex sexual behavior, desire, or identity, in combinations that vary from person to person. Among the 150 women in Laumann et al. (1994) who claimed at least one of the three dimensions of same-sex orientation (current same-sex desire, current identity as homosexual or bisexual, or same-sex behavior since age 18), Figure 1 shows that almost 60% of them stated desire only, and only 15.3% of them stated all three dimensions of same-sex orientation.

It is important to note that views of sexual identity and sexual behavior can vary significantly across cultures and among racial and ethnic groups, so it should not be assumed that a lesbian sexual orientation or

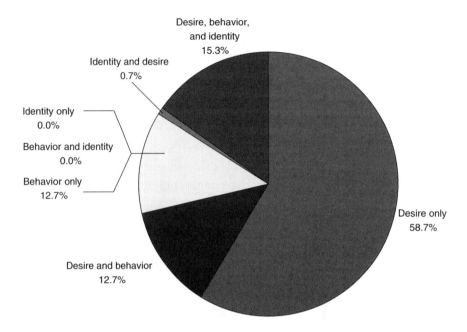

FIGURE 1 Interrelation of the different dimensions of same-sex orientation (current desire, current or past same-sex behavior, current identity as homosexual or bisexual) for 150 women (8.6% of the total 1,749) who report any adult same-sex orientation. SOURCE: Laumann et al. (1994).

identity is the same for lesbians of different racial, ethnic, or cultural backgrounds. In particular, it should not be assumed that racial and ethnic minority cultures share views of lesbian sexual orientation identical with those of the dominant culture. The committee notes that there is a dearth of research on racial and ethnic minority lesbians.

For the purposes of this report, the committee agreed that it should focus on women who have sex with or primary emotional partnerships with women. Because so little research is available about bisexual women and because the degree to which the results of research on lesbians also apply to bisexual women is unknown, the committee considers bisexual women to be a different category or subgroup of women than lesbians for the purposes of this report.

The committee strongly believes that there is no one "right" way to define "lesbian." Thus, a researcher designing a study on lesbian health should develop measures that gather information about the aspects of lesbian orientation that are relevant to the specific project at hand. Adopting this approach does not avoid the issue of establishing a lesbian definition. Rather, it builds on the need to accept the complexity of sexual orientation and the social context in which it is embedded. In essence, "lesbian" should be defined to reflect the needs of specific research studies, interventions, or programs of care within generally accepted conceptual boundaries, with a recognition of the three dimensions through which sexual orientation is most often defined: behavior, desire, and identity (see Figure 1).

The committee examined lesbian health from several different perspectives. When examined together, these various approaches can provide a more complete picture of the complexity involved in looking at lesbian health:

• **Lesbians in the larger contexts of society, the health care system, and women in general.** The contexts in which lesbians live provide a framework for understanding the complexity of their lives. For example, lesbians have historically been the target of prejudice and discrimination, both public and private, and the stigmatization of homosexuality remains widespread in our society. Although many kinds of abuse and discrimination against lesbians have been documented clearly, their impact on physical and mental health still remains to be studied. Lesbians' access to health care services may be affected by such factors as the lack of culturally competent providers[1] and the presence of homophobia[2] among providers, more limited access to health insurance because lesbians cannot share in spousal benefits, and the growing development of managed care systems that may potentially limit lesbians' access to lesbian-friendly providers. Finally, it is important to remember that lesbians confront the same kinds of health risks as do all women.

• **Health of lesbians across the life span.** All women face developmental challenges as they grow from childhood through adolescence

---

[1]Culturally competent provider refers to having a set of skills to give appropriate high-quality services to individuals from cultures different from the provider's.
[2]Meaning fear of homosexuality.

to adulthood and old age. In addition to these predictable challenges, lesbians may encounter special situations associated with their sexual orientation, such as adverse societal attitudes, family rejection, and internalized homophobia. In particular, lesbians must negotiate the process of *coming out,* or revealing their lesbian identity.

• **Specific physical and mental health concerns of lesbians, including risk and protective factors that affect these problems.** There is a great deal of speculation, with some attendant evidence, that lesbians may be at heightened risk for some health problems. Large data gaps exist, however, in knowledge about lesbian health, and the population-based information necessary to determine relative health risks of lesbians is not available. The committee examined the available data on a number of possible health risks for lesbians and reviewed what is known regarding lesbians' risk for a variety of health conditions including cancer, cardiovascular disease, sexually transmitted diseases, HIV/AIDS, and mental health and substance abuse problems. Given the limited availability of data that would allow a comparison of lesbian with heterosexual women, **the committee did not find that lesbians are at higher risk for any particular health problem simply because they have a lesbian sexual orientation**. Rather, differential risks may arise, for example, because some risk or protective factors may be more common among lesbians (e.g., higher rates of nulliparity, which is associated with increased risk for breast cancer), they may experience differential access to health care services (e.g., because of fear of coming out to health care providers), and they are exposed to stress effects of homophobia. Little is known, however, about the specific impact of these risk factors on lesbian health, and even less about any unique protective factors and how they may operate. The committee further notes that misconceptions about risk for certain health problems can negatively affect both the ability of lesbians to seek health care and the treatment itself. For example, it is important for lesbians, just as it is for heterosexual women, to obtain regular Pap tests.

Conducting research on lesbian health presents numerous challenges. First, lesbians are a population subgroup without a standard definition, and partly because of this, they are a difficult subgroup to readily identify for study. Second, lesbians constitute a small percentage of women and, in addition, are dispersed throughout the population of women, making it difficult and expensive to obtain a population based sample (or probability sample) of lesbians. Third, many in the lesbian community distrust medical research and researchers, which may result in the failure of lesbians to disclose their lesbian orientation in research studies. Fourth, there has been little funding support for research on lesbian health topics. It is not surprising, then, that methodologically rigorous large-scale studies are lacking in this area.

Although the body of research on lesbian health is growing and there are now a number of well-designed, methodologically sophisticated studies examining these issues, methodological limitations are consistently found in much of the research on lesbian health:

- **Inconsistencies in the way sexual orientation is defined, as well as the lack of standard measures, make it difficult to compare findings across studies**. Although the committee concludes that there are numerous ways to legitimately define lesbian sexual orientation in research studies, researchers have usually failed to state their definition and their reason(s) for using it.

- **The use of small nonprobability samples limits the generalizability of research results.** Most lesbian health studies have relied on nonprobability samples. In particular, many studies have used convenience samples—for example, from lesbian bars, music festivals, or gay and lesbian organizations—that are not likely to be representative of the general population of lesbians. Most samples of lesbians, furthermore, have been predominantly white, middle-class, well educated, and between 25 and 40 years old and thus are not representative of other groups of lesbians, for example, from other socioeconomic or racial and ethnic groups.

- **The lack of appropriate control or comparison groups makes it difficult to assess the health of lesbians relative to other subgroups of women**. Few studies have allowed direct comparisons between lesbians and other subgroups of women (e.g., heterosexual women) by using the same sampling strategies to identify subjects across sexual orientations and by including measures of sexual orientation.

- **The lack of longitudinal data limits an understanding of**

lesbian development and its implications for how to define and measure lesbian sexual orientation. Most existing studies portray cross sections of experience at one point in time and so cannot address compelling questions of behavior, identity, or attraction across time. Prospective, longitudinal studies are essential for understanding the vulnerability, resilience, and well-being of lesbians across their life span.

Although it can be particularly challenging to design and conduct research on lesbian health for a number of reasons (e.g., the difficulty in identifying a lesbian population subgroup from which to select a probability sample), several strategies can be used to increase the quality of research. The use of computer-assisted interviews can increase disclosure of information, and different sampling techniques can be used to produce more representative study samples.

In addition to the methodological challenges to conducting research on lesbian health, the committee identified several contextual factors that researchers must also overcome. For example, researchers studying lesbian health may experience discrimination because of the stigma associated with this population. There are relatively few researchers working on lesbian-related issues; thus, researchers can feel isolated, and students conducting lesbian-related research may lack mentors. In addition, funding for research on lesbian health has been limited and difficulties have been reported in publishing research findings.

Researchers must also establish ties with the lesbian community in order to conduct studies. Pervasive stereotypes about lesbian life, coupled with the limited visibility of this community, create the risk that researchers who fail to familiarize themselves with the community will misinterpret or misunderstand the implications of their results. This undermines the willingness of the community to provide information freely.

Research on controversial or sensitive topics such as sexual behavior, sexual orientation, or drug use is usually politically sensitive, and researchers interested in doing wide-scale studies of sexual behaviors often face political challenges to the conduct of such research. At the workshop, several possible political responses were identified that could negatively affect the future of research on lesbian health, including legislative denial of the existence of lesbians or failure to recognize lesbian health issues.

Ethical issues are also extremely important to lesbian health research. Participating in research brings potential risks for lesbians both as individual research participants and as lesbians. For example, an individual's lesbian sexual orientation might be disclosed to others (e.g., through shared use of databases if these data include identifiers), and research information could be used in some way to discriminate against or stigmatize lesbians in general. The increased need to protect confidentiality arises both because lesbians are often stigmatized and because some same-sex behaviors are illegal in some jurisdictions. The committee acknowledges these potential risks, but it also believes that significant benefits can accrue to all women from studies of lesbian health, provided that individual rights are carefully protected. These benefits include identifying areas of increased risk that need attention and identifying gaps in health care services, as well as increasing understanding of the negative impact of homophobia on health.

CONCLUSIONS

Following its broad review of what is known about lesbian health and the factors that influence it, the committee reached three major conclusions:

Conclusion 1: Additional data are required to determine if lesbians may be at higher risk for certain health problems. Further research is needed to determine the absolute and relative magnitudes of such risk and to better understand the risk and protective factors that influence lesbian health.

Conclusion 2: There are significant barriers to conducting research on lesbian health, including lack of funding, which have limited the development of more sophisticated studies, data analyses, and the publication of results.

Conclusion 3: Research on lesbian health, especially the development of more sophisticated methodologies to conduct such research, will help advance scientific knowledge that is also of benefit to other population groups, including rare or hard-to-identify population subgroups and women in general.

The committee identified several gaps and priorities for additional research, which follow:

Research Gaps and Priorities

• **Priority 1: Research is needed to better understand the physical and mental health status of lesbians and to determine whether there are health problems for which lesbians are at higher risk as well as conditions for which protective factors operate to reduce risk to health of lesbians.** There is some evidence that lesbians may be at heightened risk for some health problems. There are, however, large gaps in the knowledge about lesbian health, and the population-based data needed to determine their relative health risks are not available. It is critical that such research include consideration of the impact of socioeconomic and cultural factors on the health of lesbians.

• **Priority 2: Research is needed to better understand how to define sexual orientation in general and lesbian sexual orientation in particular and to better understand the diversity of the lesbian population.** Definitions of lesbian samples in research studies have varied widely along the multiple dimensions of sexual orientation: sexual identity, sexual behavior, and attraction or desire. Population-based data on "lesbians" are needed to better understand these dimensions of sexual orientation and the interrelationships among them, the characteristics of the population and how these characteristics interrelate with health status, and the diversity of the population.

• **Priority 3: Research is needed to identify possible barriers to access to mental and physical health care services for lesbians and ways to increase their access to these services.** It is commonly believed in the lesbian community that lesbians do not use traditional health services at the same levels as other women, although population-based data are not available to determine the severity of this problem. Nonetheless, the committee did identify a number of barriers to access to mental and physical health care services for lesbians. These include structural barriers such as the potential impact of managed care and the lack of legal recognition of relationship partners; financial barriers, which may impede access to health insurance coverage; and personal and cultural barriers, including attitudes of health care providers and the lack of cultural competency among providers for addressing the needs of lesbian clients. Developing a better understanding of the health care barriers that lesbians face could help improve access for other underserved groups as well.

RECOMMENDATIONS

The committee makes eight recommendations for improving the knowledge base on lesbian health.

Recommendation 1: Public and private funding to support research on lesbian health needs to be increased in order to enhance knowledge about risks to health and protective factors, to improve methodologies for gathering information about lesbian health, to increase understanding of the diversity of the lesbian population, and to improve lesbians' access to mental and physical health care services.

A long-term federal funding commitment to lesbian health research is needed that is responsive to the ongoing needs of the lesbian population. Foundations and other government entities are also urged to fund research on lesbian health.

Recommendation 2: Methodological research needs to be funded and conducted to improve measurement of the various dimensions of lesbian sexual orientation.

Methodological research is needed to refine the techniques available to study the full picture of lesbian health, including women of different racial and ethnic backgrounds, social classes, ages and birth cohorts, religious affiliations, and geographical locations. Although existing questions on surveys about sexual orientation are adequate for many research purposes, further work is required to improve their validity. Research is needed to determine the best ways to ask questions about lesbian sexual orientation, including the use of alternative wording and innovative technologies so as to obtain maximum disclosure. Methodological research is also needed to explore the feasibility of using different sampling techniques, by themselves or in combination, for rare or hard-to-identify population subgroups, in order to obtain a probability sample of the lesbian population subgroup.

Recommendation 3: Researchers should routinely consider including questions about sexual orientation on data collection forms in relevant studies in the behavioral and biomedical sciences to capture the full range of female experience and to increase knowledge about associations between sexual orientation and health status.

Current methodologies allow the collection of information on sexual orientation with sufficient precision to discover important relationships between orientation and other factors. Further, such questions have been used successfully in a number of research areas with different populations. Consideration should be given to including questions about sexual identity, behavior, and attraction or desire in ongoing and future federal studies, assessing multiple dimensions whenever possible and addressing the rationale for including each question. Such studies would include, for example, those in which an association between sexual orientation and health can be hypothesized or in which discrimination based on sexual orientation may result in differential access to health care services. Pilot studies are needed to test the feasibility of including these types of questions, with careful attention given to protecting confidentiality and assessing response bias and its impact on disclosure.

Researchers submitting proposals for federally funded research, whether unsolicited R01s, responses to Program Announcements, or responses to Requests for Proposals, should routinely evaluate whether or not they should include sexual orientation questions as they would other sociodemographic questions in their protocols. NIH review groups should be encouraged to consider whether or not sexual orientation should be assessed in proposed studies, and recommend inclusion of this field when it would strengthen the value of the results.

Recommendation 4: Researchers studying lesbian health should consider the full range of racial, ethnic, and socioeconomic diversity among lesbians when designing studies on lesbian health; strive to include members of the lesbian study population in the development and conduct of research; and give special attention to protecting the confidentiality and privacy of the study population.

Because there are wide social and cultural differences in the health-related stressors, risks, and protective factors to which lesbians are exposed in different social and cultural milieus, the committee recommends that studies of lesbian health include the full range of variations in race and ethnicity, social class, age, and socioeconomic status. Given the current lack of knowledge about lesbian health issues, it is imperative that researchers strive to involve members of the lesbian population being studied in the development, conduct, and dissemination of research on lesbian health. This is particularly important as a way of identifying lesbians for inclusion in research samples and securing their participation. As noted previously, the committee also urges that special attention be given to ensuring both confidentiality and the protection of human subjects in lesbian health research.

Recommendation 5: A large-scale probability survey should be funded to determine the range of expression of sexual orientation among all women and the prevalence of various risk and protective factors for health by sexual orientation.

To date no large scale probability studies on health have been conducted that collect information on sexual orientation. Conducting such a study would greatly increase knowledge about and understanding of sexual orientation in women, and improve understanding of the relationships among the dimensions of sexual orientation and health status and health behaviors.

Recommendation 6: Conferences should be held on an ongoing basis to disseminate information about the conduct and results of research on lesbian health, including the protection of human subjects.

NIH and CDC should support periodic multidisciplinary conferences on lesbian health research methods and results. The first of these conferences should take place within the next two years, with subsequent meetings to occur on a regular basis.

Given that the field of lesbian health research is still in its infancy and many researchers and members of institutional review boards are not aware of the ethical issues that need to be considered in the conduct of this research, the committee further urges that NIH in collaboration with CDC sponsor a conference on the ethical issues involved in conducting research on lesbian health, including issues related to privacy and confidentiality, future use of data, recruitment of subjects, and informed consent. This conference would be designed to inform members of institutional review boards, researchers, and members of federal review panels and should involve representatives from the lesbian community.

Recommendation 7: Federal agencies, including the National Institutes of Health and the Centers for Disease Control and Prevention, foundations, health professional associations, and academic institutions should develop and support mechanisms for broadly disseminating information and knowledge about lesbian health to health care providers, researchers, and the public.

A clearinghouse for research on lesbian health should be established to make both published and unpublished research (e.g., conference papers) available to researchers and the public; this information should be made available on-line as well.

Training programs on lesbian health and the special issues involved in working with lesbians should be developed for a wide range of providers, including pediatricians, psychologists and psychiatrists, substance abuse counselors and other treatment staff, general practitioners, obstetricians and gynecologists, and social workers. The committee also urges that health and mental health professional organizations feature discussions of lesbian health and the conduct of lesbian health research at their annual meetings.

Recommendation 8: The committee encourages development of strategies to train researchers in conducting lesbian health research at both the predoctoral and the postdoctoral levels.

Surveys of lesbians in academic settings and of graduate students indicate that individuals interested in conducting research on issues affecting lesbians face numerous barriers. In addition to the personal stigma they sometimes experience, it can be difficult to find mentors or sponsors and the funding needed to conduct the research. The availability of training funds would increase the ability of young researchers to pursue careers in lesbian health research and would enhance their skills in managing the challenges of conducting research in this area. A variety of strategies might be used to increase training opportunities for lesbian health researchers— for example, including lesbian health in the scope of pre- and postdoctoral programs in all health professions. In addition, NIH institutes should consider targeting training grants on lesbian health or including lesbian research in the scope of existing training grants. Foundations and academic institutions should also consider providing training support in this area.

REFERENCE

Laumann EO, Gagnon JH, Michael RT, Michaels S. 1994. *The Social Organization of Sexuality: Sexual Practices in the United States.* Chicago: University of Chicago Press.

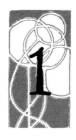

Introduction

Despite a growing but still limited body of knowledge about the prevalence, diagnosis, etiology, prevention, and treatment of health[1] problems among women in general, the health problems of some subgroups of women have continued to receive relatively little attention. Although research on lesbians has increased over the past two decades, there is still relatively little research on their health.

STUDY PROCESS AND REPORT ORGANIZATION

The Institute of Medicine (IOM) Committee on Lesbian Health Research Priorities was established in 1997 to assess the strength of the science base regarding the health problems of lesbians (i.e., women who have sex or primary emotional partnerships with women), to review methodological issues pertinent to lesbian health research, and to suggest avenues for future research. The study was funded by the National Institutes

---

[1]The committee uses the term "health" to indicate a state of complete physical, mental, and social well-being and not merely the absence of disease or infirmity. It is a positive concept emphasizing social and personal resources as well as physical capacities. The inextricable link between people and their environment constitutes the basis for a socioecological concept of health. Such a view emphasizes the interaction between individuals and their environment and the need to achieve some form of dynamic balance between the two (World Health Organization, 1998).

of Health (NIH) Office of Research on Women's Health with the Centers for Disease Control and Prevention (CDC) also contributing funding through the NIH.

Individuals appointed to the committee brought a wide range of perspectives and professional backgrounds to the workshop study, including expertise in lesbian health issues, mental and addictive disorders, breast cancer, gynecology, epidemiology, adolescence, violence against women, neuroscience, minority health, biostatistics, and sample survey methodology. Names of potential committee members were solicited from a variety of sources, including lesbian health organizations and groups with an interest in lesbian health. The committee met three times—in July, October, and November of 1997.

As part of the workshop study the committee conducted an invitational workshop on the physical and mental health concerns of lesbians and the methodological issues involved in conducting research in these areas. At the workshop, information was presented to the committee on the strength of the science base, methodological challenges in conducting research on lesbian health, and gaps in what is known about specific health problems for which lesbians may be at risk. Experts in the biomedical, behavioral, and social sciences; ethics; lesbian health; economics; and research methodology discussed the state of the field and areas in which clarification of the issues is most needed. The two-day workshop featured 21 invited speakers and included public testimony from 14 presenters (see Appendix B). Approximately 50 interested members of the public also attended the workshop and added to the discussion of the issues (see Appendix C).

To involve a wider range of people with expertise in lesbian health issues, the committee established an *ad hoc* public liaison group. The public liaison group included researchers, representatives of government and of community and national organizations, and other individuals interested in the issues. Establishment of the public liaison group reflected the committee's recognition of both the important expertise and knowledge of the issues that rests in the lesbian health community and the diversity therein. Members of the public liaison group were kept informed of the progress of the study and were invited to the public workshop and to submit testimony to the committee.

In addition to the information received through workshop presentations and public testimony, the committee identified and reviewed numerous pieces of published and unpublished literature related to lesbian health. The review included articles in the scientific literature, books, unpublished conference and meeting presentations, reports, and monographs. A listing of selected references is presented in Appendix A. The committee also received written testimony from a number of individuals and organizations unable to attend the workshop (see Appendix D). In addition, the committee's first meeting included presentations from representatives of the Gay and Lesbian Medical Association, the NIH Office of Research on Women's Health, and the CDC Office of Women's Health.

This report is the result of the information gathered by and the deliberations of the IOM Committee on Lesbian Health Research Priorities. The report reflects the committee's review and evaluation of the scientific literature on lesbian health and of the testimony presented at the workshop. Selected quotes from workshop speakers are included to more vividly illustrate for the reader some of the issues that emerged during the workshop testimonies as well as the committee's evaluation of the literature. Wherever possible reference to the published literature, surveys, workshop testimony, or other sources of information available to the committee is indicated. Statements not so referenced are those of the committee or from discussions during the workshop.

It is very important to note the limitations of this study and report. Because the study was developed and funded as a workshop study, the committee did not have the resources to undertake the in-depth level of review and analysis that is usual in a full-scale IOM study. In particular, the committee was generally unable to consider issues beyond those that were discussed at the two-day workshop, to conduct in-depth reviews of related areas (e.g., women's health in general or the effects of stress on health), to collect extensive data for analysis, to conduct detailed analyses of specific studies, or to set specific research priorities within fields of study. Nonetheless, the committee was able to conduct a broad workshop and literature review of the field and to assess the general state of knowledge across a wide range of issues for lesbian health. The review and assessment form the substance for this report.

The report is organized into five chapters. The first chapter sets the stage by describing some of the history of the workshop study, its scope, why the committee believes that lesbian health issues present an important area for attention, and how the committee defines being lesbian. Chapters 2, 3, and 4 are based largely on the workshop presentations and public testimony submitted to the committee and directly incorporate many of the presenters' remarks. Chapter 2 provides several frameworks for thinking about lesbian health: lesbians in the context of the greater society, women in general, and the health care system; lesbian health across the life span; and lesbian health with respect to specific health problems. The chapter reviews what is currently known about lesbian health, discusses the limitations of the existing literature base, and suggests health issues that should be targeted for additional research. Chapter 3 describes the methodological challenges faced by researchers studying lesbian health and discusses possible ways of dealing with them. In Chapter 4, some of the contextual barriers to conducting research on lesbian health are described. Finally, the major conclusions and recommendations of the committee are presented in Chapter 5.

WHY STUDY LESBIAN HEALTH?

Why should scientists be interested in studying lesbian health issues? Is there really any reason to think that lesbians have unique health risks or that their health risks are any different from those shared by other groups of women (e.g., heterosexual women, single women, or women who have not had children)? The committee finds several reasons why it is important and worthwhile to direct attention to the study of lesbian health issues.

• **To gain knowledge that is useful for improving the health status and health care of lesbians.** Lesbians are a subgroup of all women and so share many health risks and experiences in the health care system with women in general. For the care of lesbians to be both cost-effective and appropriate, the scope of their health problems must be better understood. In addition, knowledge of areas in which the health of lesbians differs from that of other women may provide insights to improve the health of all women.

• **To confirm beliefs and counter misconceptions that exist about the health risks to lesbians.** In the face of little empirical information there are numerous beliefs and misconceptions about the health risks of lesbians that can affect their health outcomes. These beliefs are often shared both by health care providers and by lesbians. Some of the beliefs may be true; others may be or are misconceptions. They include, for example, perceptions that lesbians do not need regular Pap tests or routine gynecological care, that lesbians do not contract HIV/AIDS, and that there is an epidemic of breast cancer in the lesbian community (Council of Scientific Affairs, 1996).

• **To identify health areas in which lesbians are at risk or tend to be at greater risk than heterosexual women or women in general.** A large body of epidemiological research has identified factors that place people at risk for health and mental health problems, with gender differences existing for many of these risk factors. However, because information on sexual orientation has not been collected in these studies, it is not possible to draw conclusions about whether lesbians in the samples differed from or were like other women with respect to these risk factors. It is possible that some factors assumed to place women at risk for or to protect them against health disorders may not be present at the same levels or operate in the same ways for lesbians. Also, as discussed later in this report, evidence from some studies suggests that lesbians may be at greater risk than other women for some health-related concerns.

In addition to facing many of the same stressors as heterosexual women, women who self-identify as lesbian may also experience stressors not commonly faced by heterosexual women (e.g., stigmatization both in and outside the health care setting). It is important to understand those factors that are unique to lesbians and their impact on lesbians' health.

DEFINING "LESBIAN"[2]

Having a clear definition of "lesbian" is critical for understanding the

---

[2]This section incorporates remarks from workshop presentations made by Meaghan Kennedy, Esther Rothblum, and Lee Badgett.

health implications of being a lesbian woman. Thus, one of the first challenges for the committee was to decide how to define the lesbian population subgroup. Popular definitions are inconsistent. Are lesbians simply women who have sex only with women? What about women whose sexual partners include both men and women? What about women whose primary affiliation is with women, but who have not engaged in sexual relationships with them?

There is no standard definition of lesbian. The term has been used to describe women who have sex with women, either exclusively or in addition to sex with men (i.e., *behavior*); women who self-identify as lesbian (i.e., *identity*); and women whose sexual preference is for women (i.e., *desire* or *attraction*). The lack of a standard definition of lesbian and of standard questions to assess who is lesbian has made it difficult to clearly define a population of lesbian women. In the research literature, definitions of lesbian also vary depending on how and where study samples were obtained.

Some researchers have included women who self-identify as bisexual in their definition of a lesbian sexual orientation; others have not. To the extent that lesbian is defined *only* by sexual activity with other women, bisexual women may then be included in the category of lesbian. If other definitions of lesbian are used, such as self-identification as lesbian or attraction to women, then a different group is identified that may or may not include women who self-identify as bisexual (see Table 3.1 for a summary of how sexual orientation has been assessed across a range of research studies).

Most of the literature reviewed by the committee was about lesbians, although it is likely that bisexual women, or even heterosexual women, have been included in some of the research samples. Much less research has been conducted that focuses specifically on bisexual women. Because so little research is available about bisexual women and the degree to which results of research about lesbians also apply to bisexual women is unknown, the committee considers bisexual women to be a different population subgroup for the purpses of this report. Nevertheless ome reported data are based on samples tdhat include both lesbian and bisexual women and, when discussed in this report, are so indicated. Some of the committee's conclusions regarding lesbians can also probably be extended to women who self-identify as bisexual, although other con-clusions cannot be generalized. For example, the methodological issues described in this report and the general difficulties of defining the popula-tion are clearly also applicable to conducting research focusing on bisexual women. However, some of the committee's other conclusions may not directly or equally apply to bisexual women (e.g., levels of risk for sexually transmitted diseases, interactions with the health care system).

It is not known how many lesbians there are in the United States, by any definition of lesbian, or the prevalence of being lesbian although estimates generally range from 2 to 10% of women (Gonsiorek and Weinrich, 1991; Laumann et al., 1994). In research, the category of les-bian is fluid with estimates of membership that vary depending on the way lesbian is defined, the current or past behavior of those sampled, and the degree to which they are willing to disclose very private and perhaps stigmatized behaviors. Lesbians do not constitute an identifiable homoge-neous population for research study. Some lesbians may belong to a com-munity of women who self-identify as lesbian and share a culture of values and norms beyond sexual behaviors. Other groups of lesbians may fear identification as lesbian, despite having emotional and sexual partnerships with women, owing to the potential stigma or negative consequence; still others may simply view their sexual behaviors as fluid within a bisexual or heterosexual identity. Diversity among lesbians also occurs along dimen-sions of race and ethnicity, socioeconomic status, age, whether or not they have children, and so on.

Racial and Ethnic Minority Groups Perspectives of Sexual Orientation

Views of sexual identity and sexual behavior can vary significantly across cultures and among racial and ethnic groups, so it should not be assumed that a lesbian sexual identity is the same for lesbians of different racial, ethnic, or cultural backgrounds (Liu and Chan, 1996). In particular, it should not be assumed that racial and ethnic minority cultures share views of lesbian sexual orientation identical with the dominant culture.

Numerous factors influence views of homosexuality among racial and ethnic minority cultures, including traditional views of family, the predominant religions within the culture, and traditional gender roles.

Other factors to consider include the time and reasons for immigration and the degree of acculturation (Greene, 1994). These factors can vary both across and within racial and ethnic minority groups. Thus, just as the attitudes of African Americans and Asians toward lesbians may differ, so may those among Latinos from Puerto Rico, Mexico, and South America. How their culture views homosexuality influences how lesbians view themselves.

Empirical data are limited on attitudes toward lesbians and the differential experiences of lesbians across cultures. However, these data can be supplemented by discussions, often by ethnic minority lesbian or gay authors, about the impact of culture on lesbian experience that illustrate the complexity involved in understanding these influences. In East Asian cultures (i.e., Chinese, Japanese, and Korean), the existence of Asian American lesbians and gay men is sometimes denied and homosexual activity is rarely disclosed to society at large (Liu and Chan, 1996). Collectivism and interdependence are highly valued, and *coming out* to family is made more difficult by the lack of a cultural framework for homosexuality. Understanding the cultural context for how homosexuality is viewed in these cultures can be greatly enhanced by taking into consideration the influences of Confucianism, Taoism, and Buddhism, religions that have influenced East Asian societies for many hundreds of years (see Table 1.1).[3]

Similar influences help form attitudes toward being lesbian in other cultural groups. For example, African-American cultures typically have a strong religious and spiritual orientation that sometimes reinforces homophobic attitudes (Savin-Williams, 1996). At the same time, traditionally strong family ties can make it less likely that a family member will be rejected because of sexual orientation, even if the family does not approve of one being lesbian (Savin-Williams, 1996). Strong gender role stereotypes are often found in Latino cultures, with distinct differences between male and female roles (Morales, 1996). Lesbian sexual orientation can be seen as threatening the cultural value of marianismo, which refers to the traditional responsibility of a woman to provide for and nurture her family

---

[3]Confucius lived from 551 to 479 B.C., Taoism was developed in the fifth century B.C., and Buddhism was first introduced into China in the first century A.D. (Liu and Chan, 1996).

TABLE 1.1 Selected Influences of Religious Heritage on Views of Homosexuality in East Asian Cultures*

Selected Influences	Cultural View of Lesbians and Gays
Confucianism—ordered relationships and roles are emphasized; children are expected to follow parents' rules and demands; concept of saving "face" is important; women are expected to be domestic, family centered, and submissive to males	A lesbian or gay sexual orientation does not fit into the Confucian order. Same-sex relationship is unfathomable and tolerated only to the extent that it does not interfere with family duties and eventual marriage.
Taoism—ancient principles of yin (the weak, passive, and negative force) and yang (the strong, active, and positive force); harmony of yin and yang is the key to happiness and the rightful order	Homosexual relationships violate the natural balance of yin and yang, which is symbolized by the marriage of male and female.
Buddhism—the key to salvation is emptying oneself of one's desires, which, after lifetimes of reincarnation, will lead to nirvana or the spiritual heaven	Following sexual desires is discouraged and will slow the path to salvation. Homosexuality is seen as resulting from pursuing one's sexual lust and is thus a reflection of impurity. However, there is no concept of homosexuality itself as a sin.

*Includes Chinese, Japanese, and Korean East Asians.
SOURCE: Liu and Chan, 1996.

and to value motherhood (Morales, 1996). Religious influences, primarily Catholicism, are likewise strong in Latino cultures. Historically, Native American cultures appear to have been relatively accepting of varied gender roles, including a lesbian sexual orientation, although contemporary attitudes, which are more influenced by the larger multicultural American culture, may be less accepting (Greene, 1994).

How the Committee Defines Lesbian

Numerous definitions of lesbian have been suggested, ranging from "someone who identifies as a lesbian" to "a woman-identified woman" or "a woman who has sex with another woman." In general, sexual orientation is most often described as including behavioral, affective (i.e., desire or attraction), and cognitive (i.e., identity) dimensions that occur along continua (Laumann et al., 1994). That is, women may exhibit differing degrees of same-sex sexual behavior, desire, or identity in combinations that vary from person to person.

Table 1.2 presents data gathered in a national study of the sexual behavior of American adults aged 18 or over (Laumann et al., 1994) and illustrates how the estimated percentage of American women who are lesbian varies depending on the definition one selects. In this sample, 3.8% of the women reported having had at least one same-sex sexual partner since puberty, 4.3% indicated that they had engaged in specific sexual activities with another woman, 7.5% reported that they currently experienced desire for a female sexual partner, and 1.4% identified themselves as homosexual or bisexual (Laumann et al., 1994).[4]

Variations in the way sexual orientation dimensions interact are also illustrated in Figure 1.1. Of the women in the survey who reported some aspect of same-sex orientation, 58.7% reported that although they found sex with another woman to be desirable, they had never had a female sexual partner and did not identify themselves as homosexual or bisexual. Nearly 13% reported that they had engaged in same-sex sexual behavior at some time since puberty, but did not identify as homosexual or lesbian and did not desire a female partner. All who reported that they identified themselves as homosexual or bisexual had engaged in same-sex behavior or found sex with a same-sex partner to be desirable. In other words, in this national sample, virtually everyone (more than 90%) who self-identified as a lesbian also reported both same-sex sexual behavior and desire for another woman. However, many women who reported desire for other women or same-sex behavior did not identify as lesbian.

The distribution of the dimensions of sexual orientation in the general population can be graphically represented in a "sexual orientation cube" (see Figure 1.2).[5] Women in cell A of the cube are clearly lesbian;

---

[4]When data from the National Health and Social Life Survey are combined with data collected in the General Social Survey since 1988, increasing the sample size to 4,827 women, 4.1% of the respondents reported having had at least one same-sex partner since they turned age 18, 2.2% reported a same-sex partner in the past five years, and 1.3% reported a same-sex partner in the past year.

[5]The example of the cube presents *one* way of measuring the dimensions of identity, behavior, and desire. There are numerous other ways of measuring these dimensions. For example, other ways of

they self-identify as homosexual, have only female sex partners, and find sex with women only to be very desirable. In contrast, those in cell B, at the opposite corner of the cube, would clearly be considered to have a quite different sexual orientation; they find sex with women not desirable, report no same-sex behavior, and self-identify as heterosexual. More difficult to categorize are those women who fall somewhere within the central portion of the cube, such as those who desire sex with women but do not identify as lesbian or engage in same-sex sexual behavior, those who identify as homosexual or bisexual but have never engaged in same-sex sexual behavior, or those women with homosexual or bisexual identity characterized by desire for both female and male partners.

As noted throughout this report, no definitive set of data containing information about sexual orientation has been developed from a large probability sample of women; thus, any attempt to represent the distribution of sexual orientation in women is subject to some distortion. The committee has analyzed data from the National Health and Social Life Survey (NHSLS) (Laumann et al., 1994) to illustrate the possible distribution of the dimensions of sexual orientation in the sexual orientation cube. These data are useful for this purpose because the study used probability sampling methods, included women from throughout the country, and included enough women in the sample (n = 1,719) to support a minimal level of analysis.[6]

For the purpose of this illustrative analysis, sexual identity was categorized as homosexual, bisexual, or heterosexual, and desire or attraction was measured by the reported appeal of same-sex behavior from not appealing to very appealing.[7] As seen later in this report, there are many

---

measuring behavior would include number of lifetime female partners or percentage of sexual events in a given time period that were with same-sex partners. Defining and measuring the dimensions of sexual orientation are discussed more fully in Chapter 3.

[6]Case-level data from female respondents in the 1995 Inter-University Consortium for Political and Social Research version of the 1992 NHSLS data set (ICPSR: Ann Arbor, Michigan) were analyzed to produce entries in the cells of the sexual orientation cube. Drs. Julie Honnold and Judith Bradford at the Virginia Commonwealth University Survey and Evaluation Research Laboratory analyzed the data on behalf of the committee. Dr. Stuart Michaels of the National Opinion Research Center, a member of the NHSLS research team, provided assistance.

[7]Sexual identity was measured by an item asking NHSLS respondents to indicate whether they considered themselves to be "heterosexual, bisexual, homosexual, or something else." Same-sex sexu-

TABLE 1.2 Percentage of Women Reporting Various Dimensions of Same-Sex (SS) Sexuality by Selected Social and Demographic Variables[a]

	Any SS Partners Since Puberty[b]	SS Activity Since Puberty[c]	Desire SS[d] Partner	Identify as Homosexual or Bisexual
Total	3.8	4.3	7.5	1.4
Age				
18–29	2.9	4.2	6.7	1.6
30–39	5.0	5.4	9.2	1.8
40–49	4.5	4.6	8.3	1.3
50–59	2.1	1.9	4.6	0.4
Marital status				
Never married	5.6	5.9	10.4	3.7
Married	2.6	2.8	5.2	0.1
Divorced, widowed, separated	4.1	5.5	9.6	1.9
Education				
Less than high school	3.3	1.8	3.3	0.4
High school graduate	1.8	2.3	5.3	0.4
Some college or vocational	3.9	5.1	7.3	1.2
College graduate	6.7	7.3	12.8	3.6
Religion				
None	9.9	11.3	15.8	4.6
Type I Protestant	2.1	2.0	5.2	0.5
Type II Protestant	2.9	3.3	5.5	0.3
Catholic	3.4	4.2	8.4	1.7

Jewish	6.9	12.5	10.3	3.4
Other	18.9	14.7	16.2	5.4
Race or ethnicity				
White	4.0	4.7	7.8	1.7
Black	3.5	2.8	7.0	0.6
Hispanic	3.8	3.5	7.6	1.1
Place of residence				
Top 12 central cities (CCs)	6.5	4.6	9.7	2.6
Next 88 CCs	5.7	7.7	7.8	1.6
Suburbs of top 12 CCs	5.7	4.1	9.0	1.9
Suburbs of next 88 CCs	3.3	4.8	9.8	1.6
Other urban areas	2.7	3.4	6.9	1.1
Rural areas	2.1	2.2	2.1	0.0

[a]Based on data gathered in the National Health and Social Life Survey ($n = 1,749$).

[b]Percentage of respondents who have had a same-sex partner at any time since puberty.

[c]Percentage of respondents who self-reported ever having engaged in specific sexual activities (e.g., oral sex, sex for pay) with another woman at any time since puberty.

[d]Percentage who reported that they were attracted to women, or that they found sex with women to be appealing, were considered to have some degree of same-sex desire.

SOURCE: Laumann et al. (1994).

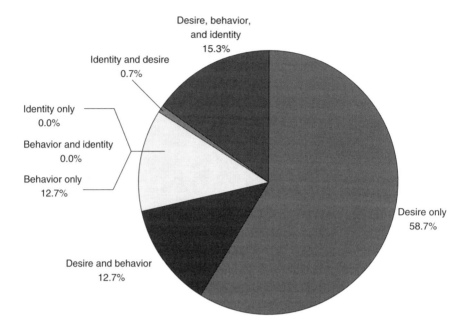

FIGURE 1.1 Interrelation of the different dimensions of same-sex orientation (current desire, current or past same-sex behavior, current identity as homosexual or bisexual) for 150 women (8.6% of the total 1,749) who report any adult same-gender orientation. SOURCE: Laumann et al. (1994).

ways in which researchers have measured same-sex behavior, usually assessing the gender of sexual partners during a certain period of time (e.g., never, ever, since age 18, during past five years). Because there were so few reports of all same-sex partners among the small number of women in this sample (*n* = 150) who reported any same-sex identity, behavior, or

al behavior was assessed with a combination of questions asking about same-gender partners and cohabitation with a same-sex partner since age 18. Of the two variables in the NHSLS measuring same-sex desire (sex of the people to whom the respondent is sexually attracted and appeal of sex with a person of the same sex), appeal was used in this analysis because it yielded a larger number of cases in the nontypical categories and, like the other variables, could be measured easily using three levels. Although these variables could be measured with a greater number of levels, only three were used to simplify visual presentation of the data and ensure that most cells were not empty. In the NHSLS report, these dimensions were analyzed dichotomously; that is, respondents were classified according to whether or not they reported same-sex behavior, desire, or identity (Laumann et al., 1994).

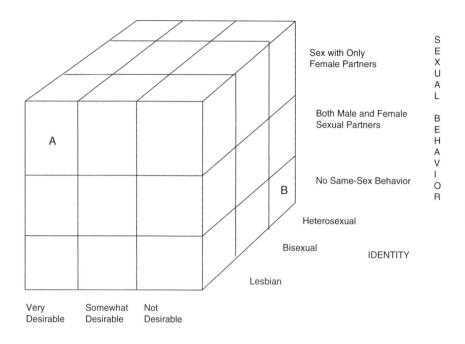

Very   Somewhat   Not
Desirable   Desirable   Desirable

DESIRABILITY OF SAME-SEX BEHAVIOR

FIGURE 1.2   Dimensions of sexual orientation: appeal by sexual behavior and identity.

attraction, the committee used a measure of history of cohabitation with a same-sex partner to assess lesbian sexual behavior from no same-sex partners to cohabitation with a same-sex partner.

Among a total of 1,719 women represented in Table 1.3,[8] 1,699 (98.8%) identified themselves as heterosexual, 9 (0.5%) as bisexual, and 11 (0.6%) as homosexual (i.e.. lesbian).[9] The great majority of self-identified heterosexuals (93.8%; n = 1,594) reported no same-sex desire or behavior (i.e., they would fall into cell B in Figure 1.2). Of the remaining 6.2%, the

---

[8]These represent the female cases for which data were available for all variables in the sexual orientation analysis.

[9]These percentages are limited by the extent to which respondents were willing to disclose their sexual identity in the context of the survey. Sexual identity was measured by an item asking NHSLS respondents to indicate whether they considered themselves to be "heterosexual, bisexual, homosexual, or something else." Issues of disclosure are discussed more extensively in Chapter 3.

TABLE 1.3 Sexual Orientation in Adult Women: Appeal and Sexual Behavior by Identity

	Appeal of Same-Sex Behavior (%)					
	Not Appealing		Somewhat Appealing		Very Appealing	
Behavior	Identify	%	Identity	%	Identity	%
Same-gender sex	A	0.2	A	0.1	A	0.1
with cohabitation	B	0.0	B	11.1	B	33.3
	C	0.0	C	0.0	C	81.8
	Total	0.2	Total	0.2	Total	0.8
Same-gender sex	A	1.6	A	0.6	A	0.2
without cohabitation	B	22.2	B	22.2	B	0.0
	C	0.0	C	0.0	C	18.2
	Total	1.7	Total	0.8	Total	0.3
No same-sex behavior	A	93.8	A	1.8	A	1.6
	B	11.1	B	0.0	B	0.0
	C	0.0	C	0.0	C	0.0
	Total	92.8	Total	1.7	Total	1.6

NOTE: Total = 1,719; A= heterosexual (n = 1,699); B = bisexual (n = 9); C = lesbian (n = 11).
SOURCE: Laumann et al., 1994.

largest numbers are found in cells representing heterosexuals who have not had a female partner but who reported that they find sex with a female to be either somewhat or very appealing, and among self-identified heterosexuals who have had a female partner but reported no same-sex desire. Although only 0.6% of the respondents self-identified as lesbian (i.e., their responses would fall into cell A in Figure 1.2), another 6.6% of the respondents reported same-sex behavior or desire. All self-identified lesbians reported that they had had a female sexual partner and that they found sex with females to be very appealing; most (81.8%, or 9 of 11) had cohabited with a female sexual partner. Self-identified bisexuals in the sample appear to occupy an intermediate position between heterosexuals and lesbians, showing less variation than heterosexuals and more than lesbians both in their sexual behavior and in how appealing they find same-sex sexual behavior.

Particularly for lesbian and bisexual women in the sample, but also for some heterosexual women, very low numbers of respondents in the cells make it inappropriate to generalize these patterns to the overall population with confidence. Further, limitations of survey research regarding the collection of valid information on sexual orientation make it likely that these data underrepresent the actual population of women who fit the study definition of lesbian (see Chapter 3).[10] Also, the results reflect an unweighted analysis even though the women in the sample differed in their probability of selection. Nonetheless, this is a useful exercise for illustrating the diversity of expression of sexual orientation in the population as well as the difficulty of grouping sexual orientation into only a few discrete categories. Additional research is needed using probability sampling techniques capable of including greater numbers of women who do *not* fit into the most common pattern of heterosexually identified women (i.e., those who have not engaged in same-sex behavior and do not find having sex with another woman appealing).

The committee strongly believes that there is no one "right" way to define who is a lesbian. For a researcher designing a study on lesbian health, the recommended course is to develop measures that gather information about the aspects of lesbian orientation that are relevant to the specific project at hand (see Chapter 3). Adopting this approach does not avoid the issue of lesbian definition. Rather, it builds on the need to accept the complexity of sexual orientation and the social context in which it is embedded. In essence, "lesbian" should be defined to meet the needs of specific research studies, interventions, or programs of care within generally accepted conceptual boundaries, with recognition of the three dimensions through which sexual orientation is most often defined: identity, attraction or desire, and behavior.

---

[10]One possible indication that respondents may be underreporting on dimensions of lesbian sexual orientation is the high percentage of self-identified lesbians who reported that they had cohabited with a female sexual partner. It may be the case that these women were most likely to have come out publicly as lesbians and thus were more likely to report their lesbian identity.

REFERENCES

Council of Scientific Affairs, American Medical Association. 1996. Health care needs of gay men and lesbians in the United States. *Journal of the American Medical Association* 275(17):1354–1359.

Gonsiorek JC, Weinrich JD. 1991. The definition and scope of sexual orientation. In: Gonsiorek JC, Weinrich JD, eds. *Homosexuality: Research Implications for Public Policy.* Newbury Park, CA: Sage Publications. Pp. 1–12.

Greene B. 1994. Ethnic-minority lesbians and gay men: Mental health and treatment issues. *Journal of Consulting and Clinical Psychology* 62(2):243–251.

Laumann EO, Gagnon JH, Michael RT, Michaels S. 1994. *The Social Organization of Sexuality: Sexual Practices in the United States.* Chicago: University of Chicago Press.

Liu P, Chan CS. 1996. Lesbian, gay, and bisexual Asian Americans and their families. In: Laird J, Green R-J eds., *Lesbians and Gays in Couples and Families: A Handbook for Therapists.* San Francisco: Jossey-Bass. Pp. 137–152.

Morales E. 1996. Gender roles among Latino gay and bisexual men: Implications for family and couple relationships. In: Laird J, Green R-J, eds. *Lesbians and Gays in Couples and Families: A Handbook for Therapists.* San Francisco: Jossey-Bass. Pp. 272–297.

Savin-Williams RC. 1996. Ethnic- and sexual-minority youth. In: Savin-Williams RC, Cohen KM, eds. *The Lives of Lesbians, Gays, and Bisexuals: Children to Adults.* Fort Worth, TX: Harcourt Brace College Publishers. Pp. 152–165.

World Health Organization. 1998. WHO Terminology Information System (WHO-TERM)—Health promotion [WWW Document]. URL http://www.who.ch/pll/ter/wt001.html#health (accessed March 11, 1998).

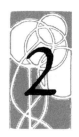

Lesbian Health Status
and Health Risks

I dentifying the physical and mental health problems for which lesbians are at higher risk is not a straightforward task. Although lesbians share many of the same health risks with women in general, a number of factors act to influence their health risks in unique ways.

In this chapter, several frameworks are presented for examining lesbian health and health risks in order to elucidate some of the unique influences on lesbian health. The first framework considers lesbians in the larger contexts of society, the health care system, and women in general. The second framework takes a developmental approach to examining the unique factors that affect lesbian health across the life span. The final framework examines specific physical and mental health concerns for lesbians, and reviews the risk and protective factors that have an impact on their risk for these problems. When examined together, these various approaches provide a more complete picture of the complexity involved in looking at lesbian health.

FRAMEWORK 1: LESBIAN HEALTH IN THE LARGER CONTEXT

Lesbian Health in the Context of Society

Historically, lesbians have been the target of prejudice and discrimination, both public and private, and the stigmatization of homosexuality remains widespread in our society (APA, 1997; Perrin, 1996). Although many kinds of abuse of and discrimination against lesbians have been clearly documented, their impact on physical and mental health remains in need of study. Until 1973 the American Psychiatric Association classified homosexuality as an illness or pathological condition. Although no longer classified as an aberrant condition, negative attitudes about gays and lesbians continue to be held by many members of the public, including health and mental health care providers (Bradford et al., 1994b; Garnets et al., 1991; Rothblum, 1994; Wolfe, 1998).

Experience with discrimination or prejudice is common among lesbians. For example, in a multisite longitudinal study of cardiovascular risk factors in black and white adults ages 25 to 37 years, 33% of the black women and 56% of the white women who reported having had at least one same-sex sexual partner reported experience with discrimination on the basis of sexual orientation (Krieger and Sidney, 1997). Eighty-five percent of the black women further reported discrimination based on race. Most of the women (89%) also reported having experienced gender discrimination.

Gay men and lesbians are also at risk of being targets of violence based on their sexual orientation or behavior. Antigay hate crimes accounted for 11.6% of the hate crime statistics collected by the Federal Bureau of Investigation (FBI) in 1996, making this the third largest category following racial hate crimes and crimes based on religion (FBI, 1996).[1] More than half of the respondents in the National Lesbian Health Care Survey (NLHCS) reported that they had been verbally attacked because they were lesbian, and 8% said that they had been physically attacked (Bradford and Ryan, 1988). Similarly, nearly half of the women surveyed in the Michigan Lesbian Health Survey (MLHS) reported having experienced a verbal attack because of their lesbian identity, and 5% reported having been physically attacked (Bybee and Roeder, 1990).

Numerous states have in place laws that negatively target gay men

---

[1]The FBI is mandated to collect data on hate crimes as part of the Uniform Crime Reporting Program, which collects data on crimes from nearly 17,000 voluntary law enforcement agency participants across the country. Of the 8,759 hate crime incidents reported to the FBI in 1996, 5,396 were motivated by racial bias, 1,401 by religion bias, 1,016 by sexual orientation bias, and 940 by ethnicity or national origin bias.

and lesbians (NGLTF, 1998; see also Table 2.1). Although some states have laws that ban discrimination on the basis of sexual orientation in employment, housing, credit, and public accommodation, many do not. Passage of such laws remains controversial. For example, in Maine where such legislation passed in 1997, voters subsequently voted to overturn the law (NGLTF, 1998). In some states, laws are in place to prohibit state and county employees from receiving domestic partner benefits. Same-sex marriage is specifically banned in 25 states and is not legal in any state. Efforts are also underway in some states to prevent same-sex couples from adopting children or serving as foster parents. Finally, numerous states ban same-sex sodomy specifically or along with opposite-sex sodomy.

> *We still have many people in many states who can be persecuted by laws, can be put out of work, and even if we have the gold standard (randomized, controlled clinical trials), they are not going to come to our studies because they do not want to be stigmatized any more than they already are.*
>
> Donna Knutson, Public Workshop, October 6–7, 1997
> Washington, D.C.

Lesbian Health in the Context of the Health Care System[2]

Lesbian health and risks to health can be examined in the context of the health care system. In other words, are there aspects of the health care system that act to reduce lesbian's access to services, thereby possibly increasing their risk of health problems? Access to health care has been defined as the timely use of personal health services to achieve the best possible health outcomes (IOM, 1993). The three primary types of barriers are (1) structural barriers (e.g., availability of services, organizational configuration of health care providers); (2) financial barriers (e.g., insurance coverage); and (3) personal and cultural barriers (e.g., attitudes of patients and providers) (IOM, 1993). The test of equal access involves

---

[2]This section incorporates portions of the workshop presentation by Jocelyn White.

TABLE 2.1 Summary of Legal Status of Lesbians and Gay Men in the United States as of May 1998

Category	Positive Policies	Negative Policies	Impact
Marriage rights	Between January and May 1998, antigay marriage bills have been blocked, defeated, or withdrawn in 4 states.	Since 1995, 28 states have enacted laws that ban legal recognition of same-sex marriages.	In states with antigay marriage laws, lesbian or gay couples who legally marry elsewhere may be denied the legal rights and responsibilities of marriage (e.g., to visit a sick spouse in the hospital or make health care decisions on her behalf). Same-sex marriages are not currently recognized in any state.
Hate crimes statutes	19 states, plus the District of Columbia, include bias crimes based on sexual orientation in their hate crime statutes.	19 states do *not* cover sexual orientation in their hate crime laws.	Hate crimes statutes that include sexual orientation make it illegal to commit crimes motivated by the victim's sexual orientation (these laws typically also include crimes motivated by race, religion, or ethnicity of the victim).

Civil rights protection	10 states have civil rights laws that include sexual orientation; at least 8 additional states have executive orders banning discrimination on the basis of sexual orientation.	In February 1998, Maine voters repealed a civil rights law, passed in 1997, that would have banned discrimination on the basis of sexual orientation; 3 states had anti-civil rights measures pending as of May 1998.	Civil rights protection for lesbians and gays prohibits discrimination with respect to such areas as employment, public accommodation, educational institutions, housing, and credit.
Sodomy	30 states do not have antisodomy laws, or existing laws have been overturned by state courts.	5 states continue to have antisodomy laws that apply to same-sex partners only; 15 states have antisodomy laws that apply to both heterosexual and same-sex couples.	Antisodomy laws make it illegal for two people of the same sex to engage in sexual activity or prohibit certain forms of sex other than heterosexual intercourse.

determining whether there are systematic differences in use and outcome among groups in society and whether these differences are the result of barriers to care. The committee finds that there is evidence that lesbians may face particular challenges in all three areas.

Structural Barriers to Health Care Access for Lesbians

Structural barriers that affect health care for lesbians include *potential* barriers presented by managed care systems and the fact that lesbian relationships are often not afforded the same legal standing as heterosexual marriages.

Managed Care. Most Americans indicate that their first choice is to see a physician in the physician's private office. Although some lesbians report that they prefer other types of providers (e.g., naturopaths, chiropractors, nurse practitioners) and to receive care in clinics, the majority report that they receive primary care from a medical doctor (Bradford et al., 1994b; Bybee and Roeder, 1990; Moran, 1996; White and Dull, 1997). Although data are not yet available to determine the impact of managed care on the quality of health care for lesbians, the committee believes that negative consequences are possible for the following reasons:

• **Limits placed on the behavior of providers by managed care organizations may introduce barriers to the effective care of lesbians.** For example, pressure to keep visits short may compromise building of trust between a provider and a lesbian patient, making it less likely that the patient will disclose her sexual orientation.

• **It is more difficult for patients to choose a lesbian-friendly medical or mental health care provider.** With unrestricted access to providers, as in fee-for-service plans, lesbians have the option of seeking out lesbian or lesbian-friendly providers. Under managed care plans, however, higher levels of coverage of health care services are generally limited to providers who are part of that particular plan. This may make it very difficult for some lesbians to identify any provider who is lesbian or lesbian-friendly, given the limited number of these providers in general. Managed care plans can reduce these barriers by identifying lesbian- or gay-friendly providers in the plan, making a concerted effort to recruit lesbian- and gay-friendly providers, and instituting cultural competency training programs to enhance the ability of their providers to serve lesbians.

• **The general lack of availability of family or household health insurance coverage for members of lesbian households makes it especially difficult for these individuals to see the same providers and enjoy family-focused care and the multiple benefits this can provide.** Although domestic partner benefits are now increasingly available through some employers, most lesbians still do not have the option of coverage under their partner's health insurance plan. If two partners are covered under different managed care plans they will have access to the same provider only if that provider is part of both plans. Additional information is needed to determine whether managed care has a differential impact on lesbian health care, and how managed care organizations can best accommodate the health care needs of lesbians.

Lack of Legal Recognition of Partners. Hospitals and health care providers do not always give the partner of a lesbian patient, or the co-parent of a lesbian's child, the same rights to visit and to access information as is provided to a heterosexual spouse. There is also, in some cases, a legal refusal to honor the lesbian partner of a patient as her health care proxy even when so designated by the patient. In the MLHS, 9% of the respondents reported that health care workers had not allowed their female partners to stay with them during treatment or see them in a treatment facility; 9% also said that providers had not included their partner in discussion about the respondent's treatment (Bybee and Roeder, 1990).

Financial Barriers to Health Care for Lesbians

Since insurance coverage is the primary gateway to health care in this country, lesbians are at a distinct disadvantage relative to married heterosexual women because of the common prohibition against spousal benefits for unmarried partners (Denenberg, 1995; Stevens, 1995). Among respondents to the NLHCS, 16% stated that they did not receive health care because it was unaffordable (Bradford and Ryan, 1988). In the MLHS, 12.3% of the lesbian sample reported that they did not have health insurance, compared to a state rate of 9.7% of Michigan women in general (Bybee and Roeder, 1990).

Although most middle-aged lesbians surveyed in the NLHCS reported good to excellent health, 27% reported that they lacked health insurance. Analysis indicated that lack of insurance may be more prevalent among lesbians with particularly serious health conditions. Lesbians without insurance were significantly more likely to report heart disease, to have Pap tests less often or never, to smoke, to have eating disorders (either overeating or undereating), and to be victims of physical and sexual abuse and antigay violence (Bradford et al., 1994a).

Personal and Cultural Barriers to Health Care Access for Lesbians

Personal and cultural barriers that affect access to care for lesbians include the lack of cultural competency among health care providers, the fear of *coming out* to providers, and the lack of lesbian focus in preventive and other health care.

Cultural Competency of Health Care Providers. Cultural competency refers to a set of skills that allows providers to give culturally appropriate high-quality services to individuals from cultures different from the providers'. These skills include understanding the culture and values of the group, the ability to communicate in the same language, and understanding the impact of group membership on health status, behavior, and attitudes. Cultural competency typically refers to providing services to people of different racial or ethnic groups. However, it also appropriately captures the skills needed to provide services effectively to lesbians. Providers who are culturally competent with respect to lesbians would be expected to understand the reasons lesbians might be reluctant to seek medical care and the impact of homophobia on the provision of services to lesbians; to be aware of the range of health problems experienced by lesbians as well as their health care risks; to avoid making heterosexual assumptions in the gathering of medical and social health information from patients; and to be willing to involve partners of lesbian patients in discussions about their health care.

Health risks and health-seeking behaviors have been found to be strongly associated with ease of communication with the primary care provider and ease of access to care (White and Dull, 1997). However, various studies of health care provider experience with and attitudes toward lesbians suggest that few physicians are knowledgeable about or sensitive to lesbian health risks or health care needs (White and Dull, 1997). Twenty percent of the women responding to the MLHS reported having encounters with health care providers who did not know anything about lesbians (Bybee and Roeder, 1990).

There is a lack of training of health care professionals in addressing the experiences and health needs specific to lesbian and gay clients, such as coming out or the lack of societal and legal recognition of relationships. A recent survey of departments of family medicine found that an average of 2.5 hours was devoted to the study of homosexuality and bisexuality across four years of medical school (Tesar and Rovi, 1998). Half (50.6%) of the 95 schools responding to the survey reported that they did not include these topics in their curricula. Diversity training in health care provider curricula can help students to recognize and overcome their biases toward clients with unfamiliar life styles, including lesbians (Black and Underwood, 1998; Robb, 1996; Robinson and Cohen, 1996).[3]

Gathering information about sexual behavior history is an essential component of good medical care. However, many physicians feel uncomfortable taking detailed sexual histories from their patients and may be particularly reluctant to inquire about same-sex behavior (Kripke et al., 1994; Merrill et al., 1990; Temple-Smith et al., 1996; Vollmer and Wells, 1989). The committee advocates training of providers to enhance their ability to discuss these issues without embarrassment and in a manner that does not threaten the patient or make her uncomfortable. Health care providers can be taught the importance of and techniques for unbiased sexual history taking (Turner et al., 1992). At the workshop, one of the

---

[3]The National Gay and Lesbian Health Association, in partnership with the Mautner Project, has produced a curriculum for training any health care provider across disciplines on addressing and removing the barriers to health care that are faced by lesbian, gay, bisexual, and transgender clients.

presenters suggested that rather than asking a woman whether she is married and what birth control she uses, it is preferable to ask whether she is in a sexual relationship, whether her partner is a man or a woman, if she and her partner are monogamous, and when she last had unprotected sex with a man (Waitkevicz, 1997). It is also important that questions be developmentally appropriate in the case of adolescents.

Homophobic Attitudes of Providers. It has been suggested that negative attitudes and responses by some health care providers may lead lesbians to avoid seeking health care (Turner et al., 1992; White and Levinson, 1993). Surveys indicate that like members of society at large, medical faculty have widely divergent views regarding homosexuality (Black and Underwood, 1998). Thus, it is not surprising that discrimination and prejudice against lesbians by both physical and mental health care providers have been reported (Denenberg, 1995; Roberts and Sorensen, 1995). This discrimination and prejudice can take many forms, including reluctance or refusal to treat, negative comments during treatment, or rough handling during examination (Smith et al., 1985).

It should be noted that a number of provider professional associations have developed statements regarding the care of people of all sexual orientations and have task forces, committees, or other initiatives in place to increase the visibility of lesbian and gay health concerns to their members and to the general public.[4]

Fear of Coming Out to Health Providers. In order to provide high-quality primary care it is important to know a patient's sexual orientation (Geddes, 1994; White and Levinson, 1995). However, the need to disclose one's sexual orientation to a health care provider can present a special barrier to care for lesbians. Fear or embarrassment may make the lesbian patient reluctant to disclose her sexuality, possibly compromising her care (Geddes, 1994; Turner et al., 1992; White and Dull, 1997).[5]

---

[4]These groups include (but are not limited to) the American Psychological Association, the American Psychiatric Association, the American Academy of Pediatrics, the American Medical Association, and the National Association of Social Workers.

[5]Of course, disclosing behaviors that might be perceived as shameful is an issue not just with respect to a person's sexual behavior, but also in other realms of sensitive or stigmatized behavior, such as drug use or domestic violence, irrespective of a patient's sexual orientation.

Someone I will call Valerie came to me last week. She said that her gynecologist had diagnosed her with cervical condyloma and she wanted my opinion about what she should do in terms of safe sex with her partner. When she asked her gynecologist this question the gynecologist said to use the condom. The gynecologist had not approached her about her sexual preference. She said, "I just don't feel comfortable coming out to my gynecologist."

J. Waitkevicz, Public Workshop, October 6–7, 1997
Washington, D.C.

Several studies have noted that the majority of lesbians (53 to 72%) do not disclose their sexual orientation to physicians when they seek medical care (Bybee and Roeder, 1990; Smith et al., 1985). Sixty percent of the women in the MLHS and 27% of respondents to the NLHCS reported experiences in which health care workers had assumed that they were heterosexual (Bradford and Ryan, 1988; Bybee and Roeder, 1990). Nonetheless, most of the respondents (61%) to the MLHS reported feeling that they could not disclose their sexual orientation to a health care provider. A much lower proportion of the respondents (16%) in the NLHCS said they would not feel comfortable letting their provider know they were lesbian.

Lack of Lesbian Focus in Preventive and Other Health Care. Primary care for women tends to be organized around reproductive health needs (Denenberg, 1995; Stevens, 1995; White and Dull, 1997). Public funding for women's health has centered on family planning and prenatal care, issues that are less salient for lesbians than for heterosexual women. Counseling for women about sexually transmitted disease, in addition, typically assumes sex with male partners. Furthermore, in many clinical environments the information forms or interviews that include questions about health history, educational materials, and insurance information assume that patients are heterosexually active (Lynch, 1993; Perrin, 1996; Rankow, 1995b; Stevens, 1995; White and Levinson, 1995). Women who are not sexually active with a man or who are not sexually active at all may thus be less likely to believe that health messages about routine care apply to them, may feel unwelcome in the health care setting, or may believe that their health needs will not be understood. In the MLHS, 60% reported that health care workers had assumed they were heterosexual (e.g., providing them with birth control supplies), and 46% reported experiences in which providers assumed they lived in a traditional family (Bybee and Roeder, 1990).

Lesbian Health in the Context of Women's Health in General

Lesbians are first of all women and thus are at risk for the same kinds of health problems as other women. The question is whether they are at the same level of risk or whether their risk is increased or decreased. Any differences in risk might be attributed to a wide range of factors: differences in health behaviors (e.g., cigarette smoking, alcohol use), differences in the stresses to which they are exposed (e.g., homophobia), or differences in the way they interact with the health care system. The major causes of death for women in general are listed in Table 2.2. This provides a backdrop for understanding the subsequent discussion of specific health concerns and the possible factors that influence a lesbian woman's risk for these problems.

For women in general, the leading cause of death is major cardiovascular disease including ischemic heart disease, cerebrovascular diseases, and atherosclerosis, followed by malignant neoplasms (cancer). Lung cancer is the most frequent cause of cancer death for women, followed by breast cancer (see Tables 2.2 and 2.3).

Additional information is presented on what is known about risk factors for various health problems among lesbians in the discussion of specific health concerns for lesbians later in this chapter.

FRAMEWORK 2: A DEVELOPMENTAL PERSPECTIVE ON LESBIAN HEALTH[6]

This section provides a brief overview of some of the developmental challenges for lesbians that can affect health across the life span. Like all

---

[6]This section incorporates portions of the workshop presentation by Donna Futterman.

TABLE 2.2 Leading Causes of Death and Age-Adjusted Death Rates (per 100,000) for Women, United States, 1995

Cause of Death (ICD-9 code)	All Women	White★	Black★
Major cardiovascular diseases (390–448)	132.9	125.1	209.5
Heart Disease (390-448)	132.9		
Heart disease (390–398, 402, 404–429)	100.4	94.9	156.3
Cerebrovascular diseases (430–438)	24.8	23.1	39.6
Atherosclerosis (440)	2.0	2.0	2.1
Malignant neoplasms (430–439)	110.4	108.9	134.1
Accidents and adverse effects (E800–E949)	17.5	17.2	20.2
Chronic obstructive pulmonary diseases and allied conditions (490–496)	17.1	17.8	12.5
Diabetes mellitus (250)	12.4	10.6	28.3
Pneumonia and influenza (480–487)	10.4	10.1	13.2
HIV infection (042–044)	5.2	2.5	24.0
Chronic liver disease and cirrhosis (571)	4.6	4.3	6.0
Suicide (E950–E959)	4.1	4.4	2.0
Homicide	4.0	2.8	11.0
Septicemia (038)	3.7	3.2	8.0
Nephritis, nephrotic syndrome, and nephrosis (580–589)	3.6	3.1	8.8

NOTE: ICD = *International Classification of Diseases,* 9th Edition.
★Data for other cultural groups not available.
SOURCE: Anderson et al., 1997.

TABLE 2.3 Cancer Incidence and Number of Deaths by Selected Sites for Women, United States, 1997

Site	Incidence	No. of Deaths
Lung	79,800	66,000
Breast	180,200	43,900
Colon and rectum	50,900	24,600
Pancreas	14,200	14,600
Ovary	26,800	14,200
Lymphoma	26,900	12,060
Leukemia	12,400	9,540
Corpus uteri (endometrium)	34,900	6,000
Cervix	14,500	4,800
All sites	596,600	265,900

SOURCE: American Cancer Society, 1997.

women, lesbians face developmental challenges as they grow from childhood through adolescence to adulthood and old age. In addition, lesbians may encounter special challenges associated with their sexual orientation, such as adverse societal attitudes, family rejection, and internalized homophobia. These special challenges can exist over the life span and depend to a considerable extent on how individual lesbians react to and manage their difference. Addressed separately is the issue of coming out, a critical stage in lesbian development that can occur during adolescence or at any time during adulthood.

Coming Out

Acknowledging a lesbian sexual orientation (i.e., coming out) has both internal and external dimensions that lesbians do not negotiate in a consistent manner. There are several descriptive models of the stages many lesbians go through during the coming-out process. One such model, proposed by Troiden, describes coming out as entailing four dimensions (Perrin, 1996; Ryan and Futterman, 1997; Sullivan, 1994; Troiden, 1988, 1989):

1. Sensitization—feel different from same-sex peers, typically before puberty;

2. Identity confusion—begin to personalize homosexuality, experience same-sex arousal and/or sexual activity, and feel inner turmoil and confusion in confronting the implications of having a homosexual identity;

3. Identity assumption—recognize homosexual identity, accept one's involvement in same-sex contacts and activities, and explore homosexual subculture; and

4. Commitment—accept homosexual identity and disclose it to others, experience same-sex intimacy, and are involved in the homosexual community.

It has been suggested that the age at which individuals come out to themselves and to others is falling (Savin-Williams and Rodriguez, 1993). Greater visibility and acceptance of homosexuality in our society may make it possible for young people to recognize and understand their feelings of same-sex attraction more readily, although additional empirical information is needed to confirm this hypothesis.

Managing the coming-out process is one way in which lesbians protect themselves against the negative consequences of living in a homophobic society. It was reported at the workshop that coming out to oneself has been shown to be a precursor to good mental health for lesbians, being associated with increased self-esteem, better psychological adjustment, greater satisfaction, and less depression or stress than experienced by lesbians or gay men who are at conflict with their identity (Savin-Williams and Rodriquez, 1993). However, coming out to others may also have negative consequences, such as being the target of discrimination or violence or experiencing rejection or physical or verbal abuse by family members or peers (Fontaine and Hammond, 1996; Morrow, 1993; Perrin, 1996; Savin-Williams, 1994; Savin-Williams and Rodriguez, 1993). Although hiding one's sexual identity or attempting to pass as heterosexual may protect adolescent lesbians from discrimination and abuse, it is also associated with increased stress, negative health and mental health outcomes, and high-risk behaviors such as substance abuse and heterosexual sexual activity, which can lead to unintended pregnancies and sexually transmitted disease (Perrin, 1996). Many lesbians thus find ways to come out to themselves and to other members of the lesbian and gay community while maintaining secrecy within their families of origin, at work, or in other areas of their lives. More information is needed about what constitutes a psychologically healthy coming-out process. This information should include focus on lesbians from racial and ethnic minority groups, lesbians of different socioeconomic status, and lesbians living in both urban and rural areas.

Ethnic minority lesbians in addition to developing their lesbian identity face the challenge of developing an identity that reflects their racial or ethnic status. This involves developing and integrating their sexual and racial identities in the context of multiple, sometimes conflicting cultures: the dominant American culture and the culture of their racial or ethnic group (or groups) of origin. Although sometimes a source of additional conflict, ethnic minority culture can also be a source of strength and support for ethnic minority lesbians (Liu and Chan, 1996; Savin-Williams, 1996). It has been suggested that having learned to handle their ethnic minority status may better equip lesbians to also handle their status as a sexual minority (Savin-Williams, 1996).

Children and Adolescent Lesbians

Very little information is available about specific developmental issues that might emerge in childhood for lesbians. There is a larger although still limited research base on homosexuality in adolescents. Little of this work, however, has focused exclusively on lesbians. Further, systematic longitudinal studies of development and adjustment are lacking (Savin-Williams and Rodriguez, 1993; Sullivan, 1994). Finally, earlier research, particularly that which focused on pathological behavior, may be of less relevance to understanding the well-being of contemporary lesbian adolescents given the contextual changes in society that have acted to increase the visibility of homosexuality and the availability of support systems for lesbian and gay youth. Nonetheless, the evidence suggests that the following issues are particularly salient for adolescent lesbians.

Development of Sexual Identity. The basic processes involved in the development of sexual orientation remain poorly understood. Although the core feelings and attractions that may form the basis of sexual orientation often emerge by early adolescence, developmental precursors have not been clearly identified for lesbian and bisexual identities (APA, 1997). Additional study is needed to better understand the processes of development involved in the acquisition and consolidation of lesbian sexual orientation and identity.

Little is known about how sexual identity develops or how the development of a homosexual sexual orientation differs between men and women. However, it does appear that awareness of sexual orientation can occur at quite young ages. In a study of 194 lesbian, gay, and bisexual youth aged 21 years or younger, respondents described their first awareness of sexual orientation as occurring at about the age of 10, with about 6 years elapsing before disclosure to another person (D'Augelli and Hershberger, 1993). There is also evidence that this awareness of identity occurs similarly in heterosexuals and lesbians. A study of 358 heterosexual, bisexual, and homosexual women reported that retrospective recall of age of first sexual or romantic attraction and of self-acknowledgment of sexual orientation was very similar in heterosexual and lesbian subjects, except for the difference in object choice (Pattatucci and Hamer, 1995). Although it has been suggested that lesbian sexual orientation may result from early sexual trauma or negative heterosexual experiences, it does not appear that sexual orientation can be largely explained by these factors (Peters and Cantrell, 1991).

Struggling with the Coming-Out Process. Developing a positive sexual identity is a normal part of adolescence. However, this can be a particularly difficult process for gay and lesbian adolescents because of pervasive societal homophobia and the lack of readily identifiable role models for positive gay or lesbian identity to help them understand what it is to be gay or lesbian (e.g., parents of gay and lesbian youth are usually heterosexual) (Ryan and Futterman, 1997; White and Levinson, 1995). Extensive social and emotional isolation (e.g., from family and peers) has been described as a frequent problem for gay and lesbian adolescents (Fontaine and Hammond, 1996; Perrin, 1996). The stigma of having homosexual feelings may make it especially difficult for gay and lesbian adolescents to seek help for their adjustment difficulties (Fontaine and Hammond, 1996; Savin-Williams, 1994).

Negotiating the coming-out process may be particularly challenging for ethnic and racial minority lesbians, who must integrate their sexual identity with their racial or ethnic identity in the face of societal homophobia and racism (Greene, 1994a, b). It has also been suggested that because members of racial and ethnic minority groups have had to learn ways of coping with racism and discrimination, when these coping mechanisms are adaptive they may provide important protective resources for coping with homophobia as well (Greene, 1994a).

It has been suggested that distress related to having a homosexual sexual orientation may lead to increased risk of attempted suicide by gay and lesbian adolescents (Fontaine and Hammond, 1996; Proctor and Groze, 1994). Although past research on lesbian and gay adolescents has generally reported rates of attempted suicide from 20 to 40%, usually based on retrospective interviews, these data have been criticized on methodological grounds. Studies have been limited by a lack of consensus on definitions of suicide attempt and sexual orientation, nonrepresentative samples, and lack of appropriate comparison groups (Muehrer, 1995). In a study of Minnesota adolescents in grades 7 through 12, which used a population-based sample, bisexual or homosexual sexual orientation was not found to be associated with increased suicide risk in girls although it was in boys (Remafedi et al., 1998). An oft-cited reference for this supposition is a background essay included in the 1989 report of the Department of Health and Human Services (DHHS) Secretary's Task Force on Youth Suicide, which suggested that gay and lesbian youth "may comprise up to thirty percent of completed youth suicides annually" (Muehrer, 1995). However, as Muehrer (1995) points out, the essay did not actually cite any published research on completed suicides. Further, there are no nationwide or statewide data on the frequency and causes of completed suicide for gays or lesbians or for the general population. Well-designed research that uses representative samples and appropriate comparison groups and considers a range of contributory factors is needed to better understand the relationships that might exist between suicide and sexual orientation.

Adult Lesbians

Many of the developmental issues that adult lesbians face are the same as those faced by other women: entering the workforce, finding a loving partner and developing a satisfying sexual life, deciding whether to have children, being a parent, and negotiating the aging process with its attendant declines in health and, for some, the death of a life partner. Little information is available, however, about how lesbians face these challenges through adulthood or about the unique challenges they may face. For example, there is a dearth of research on the practice and meaning of sexuality for lesbians throughout their life course. There is evidence that most lesbians have been heterosexually active, and this complicates retrospective and prospective analyses.

There is now a large cohort of lesbians who have lived a decade or two as "out-of-the-closet" lesbians. Midlife issues for this group are likely to be different from previous cohorts, who were less likely to publicly identify as lesbian, and to be different from those faced by heterosexual women or men. For example, many lesbians will most likely continue to struggle with issues related to balancing family and career in ways different from married heterosexual women. Little is known about specific physical and mental health concerns of lesbians as they age, particularly about lesbians of color, working-class and poor lesbians, and lesbians who are not connected to an organized lesbian community. Problems typically associated with old age may be exacerbated by poor access to health care, a problem that follows lesbians across the life span. An additional area that has received limited attention, which is discussed in greater detail below, is lesbian motherhood. Most research has focused on the effects on children of being part of a lesbian household, rather than on lesbians' decisions to become parents or the process of becoming parents.

Lesbian Motherhood.   Deciding whether or not to have children is an important and sometimes difficult issue for all women whether lesbian or heterosexual. In addition to all the usual parenting issues, lesbian parents must cope with the very real fear that they will lose their children in custody battles and other legal situations (CDC, 1997). Nonetheless, lesbians are increasingly choosing to become parents, often through donor insemination, but also through adoption and foster care (Brewaeys et al., 1995; CDC, 1997).

Research has not substantiated fears that children raised in lesbian households might grow up to be homosexual, might develop improper sex role behavior or sexual conflicts, or will have conflicts with peer groups that threaten their psychological health, self-esteem, and social relationships (Brewaeys and van Ball, 1997; Gold et al., 1994; Golombok and Tasker, 1994). There is no evidence that the development of children who have lesbian or gay parents is compromised in any significant respect relative to that of children of heterosexual parents in otherwise comparable circumstances (Golombok and Tasker, 1994; Patterson, 1992). For example, a longitudinal study of a small sample ($n = 25$) of young adults raised in lesbian families and those raised by heterosexual single mothers ($n = 21$) showed psychological well-being and evidence of comparable family identity and relationships (Tasker and Golombok, 1995). Furthermore, no differences were reported in the quality of couples' relationships or the quality of mother–child interaction between lesbian mother families and two groups of heterosexual families studied by Brewaeys et al. (1997). These researchers also reported that the quality of the interaction between the social (i.e., non-birth) mother and the child in lesbian families was superior to that between the father and the child in the two groups of heterosexual families studied.

Lesbians and other unmarried women are still sometimes refused donor insemination services.[7] One argument made against providing this service is the assertion that growing up in a lesbian household will lead to psychological difficulties for the child (Brewaeys et al., 1995; Englert, 1994; Golombok and Tasker, 1994). Research has not supported this assertion. For example, no differences in emotional and behavioral adjustment are reported for 4- to 8-year-old boys and girls ($n = 30$) conceived by donor insemination and raised in lesbian mother families, those ($n = 38$) also conceived by donor insemination but raised in heterosexual families, and those ($n = 30$) conceived conventionally and raised in a conventional heterosexual family (Brewaeys et al., 1997). Many of these studies have used small sample sizes and hence have low power to detect small differences between groups. Nonetheless, the evidence to date is consistent.

FRAMEWORK 3: A LOOK AT SPECIFIC HEALTH CONCERNS FOR LESBIANS

Lesbians may be at higher *or* lower risk of certain health problems relative to heterosexual women or women in general. These include cancer, hypertension, mental health concerns, sexually transmitted disease, HIV, and substance abuse. The data in these areas relating to lesbians are very limited. It must be further noted that there are few empirical studies of lesbian health that focus exclusively on racial and ethnic minority lesbians or that include a sizable proportion of these lesbians in their samples. Rather, most studies of lesbians have been based on samples that are primarily or exclusively white. Research that has focused on racial and

---

[7]Some lesbians use semen from known or unknown donors in the community. The use of semen from untested donors presents a possible risk of HIV infection (White, 1997).

ethnic minority women more generally has also very rarely collected information on sexual orientation (Greene and Boyd-Franklin, 1996). As a result, little is known about specific health care risks and needs of racial and ethnic minority lesbians, and significant caution must be used in generalizing the results of most lesbian health research to these populations.

Risk and Protective Factors for Lesbian Health

General Risk Factors for Health

Numerous factors have been shown to be associated with increased risk for various health problems. Table 2.4 presents general information about some of the factors that put women at higher risk of cancer. As for lesbian health research in general, information is limited on the prevalence of particular health risk factors among lesbians. The Women's Health Initiative (WHI) provides one useful source of data for looking at differences between lesbian and heterosexual women in the study in terms of certain health-related risk variables.[8]

Preliminary data from the WHI, along with limited data from other studies, indicate the following:

Smoking. In the 1996 National Household Survey on Drug Abuse, 26.7% of women reported use of cigarettes during the past month (SAMHSA, 1997). Data from the WHI indicate significant differences in cigarette smoking status depending on sexual orientation. Approximately twice as many lesbians were reported to be heavy smokers compared to heterosexual women (6.8% of lifetime lesbians and 7.4% of mature lesbians versus 3.5% of heterosexual women). Also, although almost half of the heterosexual women reported never smoking, only a third of lifetime lesbians (i.e., those whose adult lifetime partners were all women), re-

---

[8]Approximately 575 of the nearly 100,000 postmenopausal women now enrolled in the federally funded WHI clinical trial have been identified as lesbians based on data collected about sexual orientation. It must be kept in mind that the sample in the WHI may not be representative of women in the general population. It is not a probability sample; rather, women are recruited into the study using a variety of strategies. Although the WHI represents the largest study of its kind to-date, care must still be taken in generalizing the results from postmenopausal women to all women (or in the case of the lesbian subsample, to all lesbians).

TABLE 2.4 Selected Risk Factors for Cancer in Women in General

Risk Factor	Type of Cancer					
	Lung	Breast	Colorectal	Endometrial (uterine)	Cervical	Ovarian
Family history	+	+	+	+		+
Age	+	+	+	+	+	+
Smoking	+				+	
Alcohol consumption		+?				
Lack of exercise		+?	+			
Overweight		+?		+		
High-fat diet		+?	+	+		+?
Having no children		+		+		+
Use of oral contraceptives		+?		–	+?	–
Multiple male sexual partners					+	
Human papillomavirus infections					+	

NOTE: Question marks (?) indicate that there are contradictory data regarding the link between a risk factor and a particular type of cancer or that the association has not been well established; the direction of the association reported in the majority of studies is indicated.

ported never smoking, and only about a quarter (26.4%) of mature lesbians (i.e., those who reported female sexual partners only after age 50 years), reported never smoking. Reports of tobacco use by lesbians were lower in the NLHCS: 30% of the respondents reported being daily smokers, with another 11% reporting that they smoked occasionally (Bradford et al., 1994b). Current smoking levels were much lower in a more limited survey of lesbians in Oregon (11%) (White and Dull, 1997).

Overweight.   Body mass index (BMI), an indication of overweight, differed significantly between lifetime lesbians and heterosexual women in the WHI, with a greater proportion of lifetime lesbians having a BMI of more than 27 (52.3% of lifetime lesbians compared to 45.8% of heterosexual women).

History of Pregnancy.   Probability-based survey estimates are lacking for the proportion of lesbians who are mothers or the number of individuals who have lesbian mothers. Commonly cited estimates of 1 million to 5 million lesbian mothers can be criticized because the estimates are based on possibly incorrect estimates of the number of lesbians in the population (Patterson, 1998). Patterson (1998) recently analyzed data from the NHSLS (Laumann et al., 1994) to look at relationships between lesbian sexual orientation and parenthood. Women who reported having a lesbian sexual identity were least likely to have children (30%), and those reporting a heterosexual identity were most likely to have children (73%). Slightly more than half (58%) of those reporting *any* lesbian same-sex orientation (identity, behavior, or desire) indicated that they had biological children. Thus, although lesbians are less likely to report having biological children than are heterosexual women, there are still substantial numbers of lesbians who are parents, particularly if these figures include adoptive or other nonbiological parents. In the WHI sample, lesbians were much less likely to have ever been pregnant than were heterosexual women. These differences were particularly pronounced for lifetime lesbians of whom 34.1% had previously been pregnant, compared to 61.2% of the mature lesbians and 89.9% of the heterosexual women.

Use of Oral Contraceptives.   Not surprisingly, lifetime lesbians in the WHI sample were least likely to report having used oral contraceptives between the ages of 25 and 35 (only 16.7%). Approximately one-third of heterosexual women (32.0%) had used oral contraceptives during this age period as had 42.4% of mature lesbians.

Alcohol Use Among Lesbians. Reviews of lesbian health research have consistently identified alcohol abuse as a problem for which lesbians appear to be at greater risk than are heterosexual women (Cassidy and Hughes, 1997; Eliason, 1996; Haas, 1994; O'Hanlan, 1995; Rosser, 1993). Most studies, however, have had significant methodological limitations, so caution must be used in interpreting the results. Alcohol use among lesbians is described in more detail in a later section of this chapter dealing with substance abuse.

Childhood Sexual Abuse. Childhood sexual abuse has been associated with a variety of negative outcomes, including alcohol use and mental disorders such as depression (IOM, 1994). Most studies of lesbians indicate that their experiences of childhood sexual abuse are about the same as those of heterosexual women. For example, in a study of 50 lesbians admitted for substance abuse treatment in 1986–1987, Neisen and Sandall (1990) found that nearly 70% of the women reported a history of childhood sexual abuse, a rate comparable to that reported in studies of the general population of women in treatment for substance abuse (Rohsenow et al., 1988).

Like women in general, studies of lesbians who are not in treatment reveal significantly lower rates of childhood sexual abuse. Of the women surveyed in the NLHCS (Bradford et al., 1994b), 21% reported that they had been raped or attacked during childhood. Somewhat different results were obtained in a recent survey of lesbian health conducted in Chicago (Kalton, 1993). In this study, lesbians (n = 284) reported significantly higher overall rates of childhood sexual abuse (29%) than a comparison group of 134 heterosexual work colleagues (14%). However, childhood sexual abuse was not related to level of alcohol consumption or alcohol problems in either group. Finally, in a study of 523 female clients seen at a primary care health center, women who had experienced childhood sexual abuse were more likely than women who had not experienced abuse to report adult sexual experiences with women (8% versus 1%) (Lechner et al., 1993).

Unique Risk Factors for Lesbian Health

The unique effects of health-related risk factors on lesbian health as well as risk factors that may be unique to lesbians have been largely unexplored. There is little information about the social norms of lesbian communities and how these norms might have an impact on health risk. Likewise, little information is available about the risk or protective effects of lesbian relationships. One factor hypothesized to play an important role in lesbian health is stress. The possible health effects of stress for lesbians are discussed in the following section, beginning with a brief review of stress as a general risk factor for health.

The Health Impacts of Stress. Stress has been characterized as exposure to life events—either good or bad (e.g., divorce, a new job, moving to a new home, holidays, financial difficulties)—that require adaptation, or as a condition that results when an individual perceives demands as exceeding his or her ability to cope with them (Adler et al., 1994). Lesbians, like all people, experience stress as a part of everyday life. Conditions that are threatening to an individual such as physical trauma, exertion beyond one's capacity, and psychologically threatening situations activate certain physiological stress responses (see Box 2.1 for additional information about the response of the body to stress). These responses lead to adaptation and promote survival of the individual, at least in the short run (McEwen, 1998). However, such physiological responses can also have a wide range of negative impacts on health, particularly when they continue over a long term (Adler et al., 1994; McEwen, 1998).

Lesbians, similar to other stigmatized individuals, likely experience stress related to the difficulties of living in a homophobic society. Stress may result from the burden of keeping one's lesbian identity secret from family or coworkers, being excluded by physicians from making health care decisions for a gravely ill lesbian partner or, among many other factors, being the target of violence or other hate crimes. Hostility and isolation are very potent forms of stress that contribute to allostatic load by

BOX 2.1
Physiological Response to Stress

When an organism experiences stress, the body engages in a series of physiological responses. These involuntary responses are sometimes described as
"fight-or-flight" responses because they prepare an organism either to flee or to
fight when faced with real or perceived threatening situations or emergencies.
When a stimulus is perceived as threatening, the hypothalamic–pituitary–adrenal
axis, or feedback mechanism, is activated, causing the adrenal glands to release
the hormones cortisol and adrenaline.[1] Cortisol, a steroid hormone of the adrenal
cortex, promotes the redistribution of energy stores. Adrenaline, known as the
fight-or-flight hormone, is a catecholamine hormone of the adrenal medulla. The
body responds to the release of these hormones in a number of ways—for example, the pulse accelerates, respiration increases, and digestion is halted.

The process through which the body adapts to a stressful challenge and rees-
tablishes homeostasis is known as allostasis or, literally, "promoting stability
through change" (McEwen, 1998; Seeman and McEwen, 1996). In the case of
acute or short-term stress (e.g., having to stand up and give a talk before an unfamiliar audience), the two physiological response systems involved in allostasis are
turned on, leading the organism to adapt to the stress and survive the potential
crisis. However, many people are prone to worry and to experience anxiety, and
therefore experience stress for much longer periods of time, resulting in repeated
or continued activation of the stress response. This may come about when there
are too many stressful events, when the cortisol and adrenaline systems fail to
shut off after the stress is over, or when they fail to habituate to chronic stress. In
any of these cases, the result is the same, namely, the body is overexposed to its
own stress hormones over weeks, months, and even years.

The body pays a price for overexposure to stress hormones. For example,
repeated stress elevates blood pressure and can lead to hypertension; the ste-
roids produced during chronic stress can lead to the depositing of abdominal fat,
which—when combined with elevated blood pressure—accelerates atherosclerosis in some people, and elevated cortisol in people with depressive illness promotes calcium loss from bone as well as muscular weakening. Elevated cortisol
and the neural activity associated with stress can also cause nerve cells in the
hippocampal region[2] of the brain to atrophy, resulting in some cognitive impair-
ment; in the extreme, atrophy of nerve cells can lead to permanent cell loss and
permanent damage (McEwen, 1998).

Thus, the same processes of allostasis that promote adaptation can also exac-
erbate disease processes when they become inefficient or overly active (McEwen,
1998; Seeman and McEwen, 1996).

---

[1]Hormones are substances secreted by the body that help to regulate the functioning of tissues or organs.
[2]The hippocampus is a region of the brain that plays a central role in memory
processes.

leading to elevated levels of the stress hormones (McEwen, 1998; Powch and Houston, 1996). Although the precise health effects of stress on lesbians have not yet been examined systematically, some hypotheses can be made about their possible health risk based on information about both the stress effects of discrimination on other groups and the stress effects of socioeconomic status.[9] It can be hypothesized that lesbians who experience such forms of psychosocial stress sustain negative effects similar to those of other groups that experience discrimination.

It can also be hypothesized that stress effects may be greatest for lesbians who are subject to multiple forms of discrimination, for example, lesbians who are also members of racial or ethnic minority groups. In addition to experiencing racism encountered by members of racial and ethnic minority groups in general, minority lesbians can also encounter racism in the lesbian community (Savin-Williams, 1996). Racism may thus compound the negative effects that homophobia potentially has on health. The combination of homophobia, racism, and sex-based discrimination has been referred to as being in "triple jeopardy" (Greene, 1994b; Greene and Boyd-Franklin, 1996).

A study of depressive distress in a nationally recruited homosexually active sample of African-American men and women showed that lesbians and bisexual women in the sample exhibited higher levels of distress than gay men, except for those with HIV infection (Cochran and Mays, 1994). The authors suggest that individuals who carry multiple lower social statuses (i.e., being lesbian, being a racial or ethnic minority, and being female) may be particularly at risk for stress-induced depression.

Racial discrimination has been found to be a potent source of stress and to be associated with stress-related negative health effects (Krieger and Sidney, 1996). To assess the role of racial discrimination in explaining disparities in elevated blood pressure, a common reaction of people who

---

[9]A very notable and important exception to the lack of research in this area is a recent study by Krieger and Sidney (1997), which examined associations between self-reported experiences of discrimination based on sexual orientation among black and white women and men participating in a longitudinal multisite study of cardiovascular risk factors. Meaningful analyses of systolic blood pressure in relation to reported experiences of discrimination were precluded by the small number of participants for whom data were available, particularly black women and men (Krieger and Sidney, 1997).

experience psychosocial stress, Krieger and Sidney (1996) examined associations between blood pressure and self-reported experiences of racial discrimination and unfair treatment in a multisite, multiethnic sample.[10] In this study, black individuals who reported that they internalized experiences of discrimination (e.g., accepted these as a fact of life or kept to themselves) had higher blood pressure than both white individuals and black individuals who reacted to experiences of discrimination when they occurred (e.g., did something or talked to others). The researchers concluded that racial discrimination helps to shape patterns of blood pressure among black individuals in the United States and to account for some of the differences in blood pressure observed between white individuals and black individuals.

Socioeconomic status (SES) embodies aspects of stress resulting from different living and working environments as well as economic factors and physical security. There are gradients of health that occur across the full socioeconomic spectrum, and SES, particularly income inequality, has been shown to be predictive of health status (Adler et al., 1993; Kawachi and Kennedy, 1997). These SES relationships are manifest as gradients of mortality and morbidity related to cardiovascular disease and abdominal obesity, with the poorest and least well educated having significantly poorer health and shorter life spans, on average, and the wealthiest and best-educated having significantly better health and longer life spans than those in the middle of the gradient.

Individuals of lower SES are more likely to encounter negative life events than those at higher SES levels and tend to have fewer social and psychological resources for coping with stress (Adler et al., 1994). Both factors can make these individuals more vulnerable to stress. For example, it has been demonstrated that characteristics of the social environment, in particular the presence of social relationships, influence patterns of response to stressful stimuli (Seeman and McEwen, 1996). For lesbians at lower socioeconomic levels the negative effects of stress associated with discrimination may be compounded.

---

[10]Data were collected as part of the Coronary Artery Risk Development in Young Adults (CARDIA) study, which was a multisite community-based study designed to investigate the evolution of cardiovascular risk factors (Krieger and Sidney, 1996). Participants were 25 to 37 years of age.

Protective Factors for Lesbian Health

A variety of factors can act to protect individuals from negative outcomes, including a close relationship with a responsive and accepting parent, attachment to external support systems such as schools or churches, and having well-developed social support systems (IOM, 1994). Although research is quite limited, some factors have been suggested to be protective of lesbian health. One of the suggested protective factors is involvement in the lesbian community (White and Levinson, 1993). Although midlife lesbians responding to the NLHCS reported high levels of stress, most reported that they relied on the lesbian community and on lesbian and gay male friends for support and socialization and reported overall satisfaction with their lives (Bradford and Ryan, 1988).

Strong family ties can also have protective effects. Additional research is needed on the relationships between lesbians and members of their families and on the influences of these relationships on mental health. Rejection and disapproval from family members may be major stressors for lesbians, just as acceptance and support may be protective factors (APA, 1997).

Specific Health Concerns for Lesbians

Several potential health concerns for lesbians are discussed in this section because there is some empirical evidence to support the belief that lesbians are at higher risk for a particular problem, because there are widely held assumptions of greater risk, or because possible misconceptions about lesbians' risk for a problem have important implications for health care and health-seeking behavior. In reviewing information about the health concerns of lesbians it is important to keep in mind the factors that have been presented thus far; that is, the risk for particular health problems must be considered in the larger contexts of women's health, the health care system, and society. Particular health problems become more salient at different points along the developmental pathway, and there are both risk and protective factors that affect health.

Cancer and Lesbians[11]

The most common form of cancer in women in the United States is breast cancer, followed by lung cancer, cancer of the colon and rectum, uterine cancer, and ovarian cancer (see Table 2.3). The order of frequency of diagnosis of particular cancers varies somewhat across racial and ethnic groups. For example, although breast cancer is the most commonly diagnosed cancer for both white and black women, the second most frequently diagnosed cancer for black women is cancer of the colon and rectum and for white women lung cancer (American Cancer Society, 1997).

Risk factors have been identified that put women at greater risk for particular cancers (see Table 2.4). For most cancers, risk increases with age or with a family history of that type of cancer. In addition, however, there are behavioral factors, such as smoking, consumption of alcohol, or sexual history, that can increase the risk of cancer. In some cases, the association between a type of cancer and a risk factor is clear and well established (e.g., the link between smoking and lung cancer), in other cases, the data are less clear.

Much attention has been paid to possible increased risk of cancer among lesbians, particularly with respect to breast cancer. The assumption of higher risk for lesbians is based primarily on data from various studies suggesting that certain cancer risk factors occur at higher levels or with greater frequency in lesbians (Turner et al., 1992; White and Levinson, 1993). These factors include higher rates of smoking, alcohol use, poor diet, greater BMI, and differential rates of hormone exposure associated with less use of oral contraceptives and the lower likelihood of bearing children (Rankow, 1995a). To date, however, there are no epidemiological studies supporting a conclusion that lesbians are at increased risk for breast or other cancers.

There are several reasons for studying cancer among lesbians. For example, compared to heterosexual women, lesbians may have differences in risk factors, differences in prevalence of risk factors for each of the cancers, and differences in the way that health care is received (e.g., how

---

[11]This section is based largely on the workshop presentation by Dr. Deborah Bowen.

they relate to their health care provider, how the provider relates to them).

Breast Cancer.   Excluding skin cancers, breast cancer is the most common cancer among women. According to the National Cancer Institute, approximately one in eight women in the United States will develop breast cancer during her lifetime with most cases occurring after the age of 50 (NCI, 1997). There is some evidence that the prevalence of certain risk factors for breast cancer may be higher among lesbians. Some studies have suggested that lesbians have higher rates of alcohol consumption and being overweight and that they are less likely to have had children than are women in general. However, it is important to state that the appropriate epidemiological research has yet to be done to determine whether lesbians are at greater risk for breast cancer. Thus, the committee concludes that insufficient data are now available to determine whether lesbians have a higher risk for breast cancer than women in general.

Whether or not lesbians are at higher risk of breast cancer than heterosexual women, there is a common perception in the lesbian community that they are. In a controlled clinical trial of breast cancer risk, when lifetime risk of breast cancer was calculated for a sample of lesbians and for a general sample of women, women in the general sample were found to have a 13% mean risk of breast cancer by age 80 whereas women in the lesbian sample were found to have an 11% mean risk (Bowen et al., 1997). Both groups of women, however, perceived their risk to be substantially higher, with lesbians believing that they had a 36% mean lifetime risk and women in the general sample believing they had a 50% mean lifetime risk of breast cancer (i.e., by age 80). When only women with a family history of breast cancer were included in the sample, the perceived lifetime risk was nearly identical for lesbians and the general sample. From this and other studies it is apparent that women (both lesbian and heterosexual) tend to believe that their risk of breast cancer is much higher than it really is. These misperceptions of risk can have an impact on whether or not one gets a regular mammogram and on one's quality of life (e.g., fear of breast cancer causing increased stress).

Cervical Cancer. Cervical cancer accounts for 6% of all cancers in women and is the ninth most deadly cancer for women in the United States (American Cancer Society, 1997). Cervical cancer risk in women in general is highly associated with sexual behavior (e.g., multiple male sexual partners or partners who have had multiple sex partners, early age at first intercourse, unprotected sex) and with the presence of certain genotypes of human papillomavirus (HPV), a common sexually transmitted infectious virus (Price et al., 1996). HPV can cause cervical warts, and some HPV types have a high association with the development of cervical cancers, although after many years of HPV infection. Changes in the cells of the cervix resulting from HPV infection, including early stages of cervical neoplasia as evidenced by squamous intraepithelial neoplasia, can be detected by the Pap test. The Pap test is the most important screening tool used to diagnose and, through subsequent treatment of epithelial abnormalities, to prevent the development of invasive cervical cancer. Early detection of cervical epithelial cell abnormalities through Pap tests has greatly reduced the number of deaths resulting from cervical cancer over the past 20 years.

The important association between female sexual behavior with men and risk of cervical cancer might seem to imply that lesbians are not at meaningful risk for cervical cancer. However, lesbians clearly remain at risk for cervical cancer, albeit probably at less risk than women in general, because the great majority of lesbians report a history of having had heterosexual intercourse (Bevier et al., 1995; Bybee and Roeder, 1990; Ferris et al., 1996; Gómez, 1994; Price et al., 1996; Skinner et al., 1996; White, 1997). Cervical neoplasia associated with HPV infection has been detected in lesbians even in the absence of prior reported sex with men (Marrazzo et al., in press; O'Hanlan and Crum, 1996; Robertson and Schachter, 1981). Genital warts have also been detected in lesbians (Marrazzo et al., in press), including women who deny having had sex with men (Edwards and Thin, 1990).

Some data suggest that lesbians may have routine Pap tests less frequently than is currently recommended (Robertson and Schachter, 1981; Stevens, 1992). For example, 23% of the respondents in the NLHCS reported that their last Pap test was more than two years ago (Bradford and Ryan, 1988), and the mean interval since their last Pap test was 34 months in a sample of 104 lesbians attending a lesbian health clinic in Washington, DC (Biddle, 1993). Evidence is mixed, however, regarding whether lesbians differ from heterosexual women in their frequency of Pap test screening. Some studies (e.g., the WHI; Price et al., 1996) have found no significant differences between heterosexuals and lesbians in Pap test screening behavior. A randomized controlled trial of counseling for breast cancer risk, however, which included more economically disadvantaged women, found that lesbians were less likely than women in general to get a Pap test at least once a year (Bowen et al., 1997). In another community study, the mean interval between routine Pap smears was longer for lesbians than for age-matched heterosexual women attending the same clinic (21 months versus 8 months, Marrazzo et al., 1996a). Lesbians without prior male sexual partners may also be less likely to get Pap tests. More than half (57%) of the women in that study who had never had sex with a male partner reported having two or fewer routine Pap smears in the preceding five years compared to 21% of the women with male partners during that time ($p \leq .01$). Nevertheless, whether Pap test screening is indeed less frequent among lesbians, particularly those who have not had sex with men, requires further investigation. Conditions that could contribute to less frequent Pap test screening, including perception of low risk for cervical cancer or barriers to health care, need to be defined.

Other Cancers. Less information is available on other cancers among lesbians. If it is indeed true that lesbians have higher rates of smoking, then they are likely at increased risk of lung cancer. However, data are mixed on the prevalence of smoking in the lesbian population as well as on the patterns of smoking. There is some evidence that lesbians tend to have a higher BMI; if this is accompanied by a high-fat diet, they may be at greater risk for colorectal, ovarian, or endometrial cancers. Because lesbians are less likely to have had children and less likely to use oral contraceptives, they may be at increased risk for endometrial or ovarian cancers. However, because the necessary epidemiological data on these health risk factors among lesbians are not available at this point, it is not possible to determine whether lesbians are at increased risk for these cancers.

Cardiovascular Disease and Lesbians

Cardiovascular diseases—heart disease, stroke, and atherosclerosis—represent the leading cause of death for women in general. Risk factors for heart disease include cigarette smoking, high blood pressure (hypertension), high blood cholesterol, excessive weight, use of oral contraceptives, and physical inactivity (NHLBI, 1997). Although stress has been shown to be a possible risk factor for cardiovascular disease in men, this connection has not yet been demonstrated in women. Moderate consumption of alcohol (one or two drinks per day) may have some protective effects against cardiovascular disease as does the use of hormone replacement therapy for menopausal women.

There are no population-based data on cardiovascular disease among lesbians or on the factors that increase their risk for cardiovascular disease. There is some evidence that lesbians may have higher rates of smoking and higher BMI, two risk factors for cardiovascular disease. On the other hand, lesbians are less likely to use oral contraceptives, which may lower their risk for cardiovascular disease. Based on currently available data, the committee concludes that it is not possible to determine whether lesbians are indeed at higher risk for cardiovascular disease than women in general.

Mental Health Issues for Lesbians[12]

The most common mental disorders experienced by women in general are anxiety disorders. Data from the National Comorbidity Survey, the first survey to administer a structured psychiatric interview to a probability sample in the United States, indicate that 30.5% of the women surveyed reported experiencing an anxiety disorder at some time in their lives (usually social phobia or simple phobia); 22.6% reported such a disorder during the past year (Kessler et al., 1994). The next most common category of mental disorders experienced by women in general is affective disorders, with depression being most commonly reported. In the National Comorbidity Survey, 23.9% of the women surveyed reported expe-

---

[12]This section is based largely on the workshop presentation by Dr. Margery Sved and the public testimony of the American Psychological Association, presented by Dr. Charlotte Patterson.

riencing an affective disorder at some time; 14.1% reported experiencing such an episode during the past 12 months. A previous episode of major depression was reported by 21.3% of the women; 12.9% reported experiencing a major depressive episode during the past year.

Very little is known about the prevalence and incidence of depression, anxiety disorders, psychotic disorders, dissociative disorders, and personality disorders in lesbians (Rothblum, 1994; Trippet, 1994).[13] In general, studies have not found differences in the psychological adjustment of nonclinical samples of lesbians and other women (Rothblum, 1994). Although there is, in general, no reason to expect that most major mental illnesses occur more or less often in lesbians than in heterosexual women, except perhaps owing to the experience of discrimination, not enough information is available to draw definitive conclusions.

About three-quarters of all respondents in the NLHCS reported participating in counseling, indicating that they experienced or sought care for the same kinds of mental health issues experienced by women in general (Bradford et al., 1994b).[14] These respondents reported depression; anxiety; relationship problems; problems with children, parents, or other family members; work-related problems; substance abuse; loneliness; losses; past or present physical or sexual abuse; other trauma; and major mental illnesses such as bipolar disorder and schizophrenia. However, whether any of these issues, themes, or illnesses occur more often or differently in lesbians than in other women is not known.

The reported rates of depression for lesbians responding to the NLHCS appear to be somewhat similar to those reported for heterosexual women.[15] More than half of the respondents reported thoughts of suicide

---

[13]One review of six major psychological counseling journals published from 1978 to 1989 found that only 43 of 6,661 articles adressed gay and lesbian issues (Buhrke et al., 1992).

[14]The NLHCS (Bradford and Ryan, 1988) remains the most comprehensive study of the health and mental health of lesbians in the United States. However, although the survey provided valuable information about the health of lesbians, it did not compare lesbians to all women or to heterosexual women.

[15]In the National Comorbidity Study, 21.3% of women surveyed were reported to have experienced a major depressive episode at some time during their lives, with 12.9% having experienced a major depressive episode during the previous 12 months (Kessler et al., 1994). In the NLHCS, 37% of the respondents reported that they had experienced a "long depression or sadness" at some point in the past (a broader category than "major depressive episode"), and 11% indicated that they were currently experiencing such feelings.

at some time, and 18% reported that they had attempted suicide. Although these numbers appear high, because there is no reliable source of information about suicide attempts by women in the general population, it is not possible to determine how such figures compare to a similar population of heterosexual women (Muehrer, 1995). The rates of physical abuse, sexual abuse, and incest do not appear to be significantly different from similar reports for all women (Bradford et al., 1994b).

Most of the more recent literature presents data on mental health issues and mental health treatment in self-identified lesbians. As with other areas of lesbian health research, research samples have primarily included self-identified lesbians who are white, middle class, in college or college-educated, urban or suburban, and young to middle aged. Little information is available regarding mental health issues for other groups of lesbians, such as racial and ethnic minority lesbians, poor or working-class lesbians, older lesbians, or lesbians living in rural areas.

Information about the access to or utilization of mental health care services by lesbian women is limited. Although high percentages of lesbians in some surveys have reported that they have used mental health services, the results are not based on probability samples (Bradford et al., 1994b). Additional research is needed to determine the generalizability of these findings. Research is also needed to examine the experiences that lesbians have in mental health care settings and the effectiveness of various therapeutic approaches with lesbians.

Sexually Transmitted Diseases Among Lesbians[16]

The high levels of sexually transmitted diseases (STDs) in the United States have been described as a hidden epidemic (IOM, 1997). In 1995, for example, nearly 384,000 women were reported to have chlamydia, nearly 189,000 to have gonorrhea, and more than 34,000 to have syphilis (CDC, 1996). STDs can have numerous negative outcomes for women, including cervical cancer, chronic pelvic pain, infertility, and ectopic pregnancy (IOM, 1997).

---

[16]This section is adapted from written testimony submitted by Dr. Jeanne Marrazzo and includes comments from the workshop presentation of Dr. Jonathan Zenilman.

The risk of developing STDs depends on several factors. Women are particularly at risk in heterosexual vaginal and rectal intercourse because with penile insertion and ejaculation, the amount of bacteria or virus that is transmitted is much higher than in other kinds of sexual activity. Another important factor is the number of sexual partners. The more partners one has and the more contacts with each individual partner, the higher the risk. Many STDs are transmitted more readily from men to women than from women to men (IOM, 1997).

Although it is well known that women can acquire STDs from male sex partners, the risk of STD transmission between female partners is unclear. Guidelines for safe sex for lesbians are lacking (Denenberg, 1995; Rankow, 1995a). Attempts to use national or local surveillance data to estimate the risk of STD transmission between women are limited by the fact that many risk classification schemes have either excluded same-gender sex among women or subsumed it under a hierarchy of other behaviors viewed as higher risk (Chu et al., 1990, 1992). Moreover, few if any state or local STD reporting systems routinely collect and analyze information on same-sex behavior among women. Nonetheless, lesbians are often perceived to be at very minimal risk for STD. This perception has three apparent sources:

1. Previous Reports of Low Prevalence. A few studies have reported low prevalence of STD among women who report having sex with women (Robertson and Schachter, 1981) and no risk of transmission of HIV between female sex partners (Raiteri et al., 1994b).[17] However, these studies evaluated small numbers of women and did not employ newer diagnostic tests including amplified DNA probes and serologic techniques, particularly for viral STDs. They also did not provide complete information on sexual behaviors. The single prospective study evaluating risk of HIV transmission in HIV-discordant female couples, moreover, was limited by a short follow-up period of six months (Raiteri et al., 1994b; Reynolds, 1994).

2. Assumptions About Sexual Practices Between Women. It is often presumed that lesbian sex does not involve contact between mu-

---

[17]Some studies included women who reported having had sex with men as well as women.

cous membranes, such as that which occurs during vaginal–penile sex, implying a low risk of bacterial STD transmission for anatomic reasons. In fact, data on the specific sexual practices of lesbians are extremely limited and there are no large-scale contemporary studies based on probability samples.[18] Limited data on sexual practices among lesbians are presented in Table 2.5. Although caution should be used in generalizing these data, they do give an indication of the range of sexual practices among lesbians.

The potential exists for transmission of some STDs that require only skin contact (e.g., herpesvirus), and the sharing of vaginal secretions via hands or sex toys could introduce pathogens into the vagina. Perhaps of greater importance, most lesbians have had sex with men, and an estimated 21 to 30% continue to have male sex partners (Einhorn and Polgar, 1994; Ferris et al., 1996; O'Hanlan and Crum, 1996). It is unknown whether the male sexual partners of these women are more or less likely to be infected with one or more STDs. Acquisition of chronic STDs from male partners thus presumably occurs with the same frequency for these women as for heterosexual women. Because viral infections such as herpes and HPV can result from previous exposure unrelated to current sexual activity, it is particularly important to consider the sex of past sexual partners.

3. Assumptions About the Course of Lesbian Relationships. There are numerous assumptions about lesbian relationships and lesbian sexual networks that contribute to the perception that lesbians are at low risk for STD. These include the perception that rates of partner change are low, that monogamous lesbian relationships tend to be long-lasting, and that concurrent sexual relationships outside of monogamous relationships are less common than in heterosexual or male homosexual populations (Kennedy et al., 1995).

Classical STDs, such as syphilis, gonorrhea, and chlamydia, are indeed rare in women who have sex *only* with women, in part because of

---

[18]Although the NHSLS (Laumann et al., 1994) is based on a national probability sample, the sample of lesbians in the study is small, precluding detailed analyses of the data on sexual practices because of the small number of respondents reporting behaviors across categories.

sexual behavior and in part because of issues related to transmission efficiency. A more complete understanding of the specific sexual behaviors of lesbians is needed because there are few data on the sexual activities in which lesbians actually engage.

Several studies have examined genital infection with HPV and bacterial vaginosis[19] (BV) among women who have sex with women. Work by Marrazzo and her colleagues and others suggests that these infections are common among lesbians, including those who have never had sex with men (Marrazzo et al., in press). The prevalence of BV among lesbians has been reported to be 18 to 36% (Berger et al., 1995; Edwards and Thin, 1990; Marrazzo et al.,1996a, b), higher than the 16% prevalence seen in 10,397 pregnant women evaluated in the Vaginal Infections in Pregnancy study (Hillier et al., 1995). A study of 101 lesbians, none of whom had had sex with men during the preceding year, found BV prevalence to be 29%. In that study, 73% of index subjects with BV had partners with BV, whereas BV was documented in only 10% of partners of women without BV. A study conducted in a London genitourinary medicine clinic compared 241 lesbians and 241 matched heterosexual controls and found higher rates of BV in lesbians.

In a recent pilot study to examine the prevalence of STD and cervical neoplasia in a group of lesbians recruited through community advertisements, nearly one-third of the 149 study subjects had experienced at least one episode of BV (Marrazzo et al., in press). Eighteen subjects (18%) had BV at the time of study evaluation. Of the 17 who had had sex with men, the time from last sex with a male partner was greater than three months for 16 of them (91%). All subjects with BV reported receptive oral sex and mutual digital–vaginal sex.

There are no specific data about the prevalence of STDs in lesbian teenagers. With the recent upsurge in herpes type 2 infections among adolescent women and the possibility of transmission by orogenital and hand–genital contact, however, lesbian youth may be at high risk.

---

[19]Bacterial vaginosis is an ecological disturbance in the bacterial microflora in the vagina that has been implicated in numerous upper genital tract conditions, including pelvic inflammatory disease and adverse outcomes of pregnancy (Eschenbach, 1993; Hillier et al., 1995).

TABLE 2.5 Sexual Practices in Selected Samples of Lesbians

Study	Focus of Study	Reported Sexual Practices
Michigan Lesbian Health Survey (Bybee and Roeder, 1990)	General health and HIV risk of lesbians across the state of Michigan (*n* = 1,681)	During past 3 years: Oral sex during menstrual periods (38.1%) Shared sex toy with possible exchange of body fluids (25.6%) Oral-anal sex (16.9%) Anal penetration with bleeding or injury (2.4%) Taken urine or feces into mouth or vagina (1.7%)
National Health and Social Life Survey (Laumann et al., 1994)	Sexual behaviors and practices of Americans (*n* = 3,432 total men and women; *n* = 1,749 women; *n* = 150 women reporting any same-gender sexuality)	Sexual practices of women who reported *any* same-gender sexuality, behavior, or desire: Masturbation weekly or more frequently during past year (49.6%) Active oral sex ever (26.7%) Receptive oral sex ever (34.6%) Sexual practices among women who reported any same-sex partners *in past 5 years*: Masturbation weekly or more frequently during past year (20.0%) Active oral sex ever (71.4%) Receptive oral sex ever (82.1%)
Raiteri et al., 1994b	HIV seroprevalence, behavioral risks, and attitude toward HIV infection among self-identified lesbians in Turin, Italy (*n* = 181)	Sexual practices, 1991–1992: Deep kissing, breast fondling, mutual masturbation (100.0%) Cunnilingus (100.0%) Sex during menses (95.1%) Reciprocal exchange of sexual devices (77.6%) Anal manipulation (46.1%) Group sex (4.2%)

TABLE 2.5 Continued

Study	Focus of Study	Reported Sexual Practices
Russell et al., 1995	Presence of sexually transmitted pharyngeal bacteria and carriage rate in sexually active adults attending a genitourinary clinic (*n* = 492 heterosexual women; *n* = 41 lesbians; *n* = 9 bisexual women; *n* = 586 men)	Following types of orogenital contact in past 2 weeks: Any oral contact (44%) Vulva/vagina contact 37%) Vulva/vagina and anus contact (7%) Anus only contact (0%)

HIV and Lesbians

Among the 85,500 U.S. female AIDS cases reported to the CDC as of December 1996 (CDC, 1997), 45% were attributed to injection drug use, 38% to heterosexual contact, and 17% to infection by contaminated blood products or an undetermined route of infection. Undistinguished within these cases of women with AIDS are women who report sexual behaviors with women and women who self-identify as lesbian (Mays, 1996). The prevalence of HIV infection among women who have sex with women (WSW)[20] is unknown owing to the methodological barriers in attaining representative samples of these women (Kennedy et al., 1995) and the lack of HIV research studies targeting these populations. The few studies of WSW that assess HIV seroprevalence provide differing estimates of HIV infection rates, possibly attributable to the type of WSW populations sampled. Most studies, however, suggest higher HIV seroprevalence among WSW compared to exclusively heterosexual women (Bevier et al., 1995; Cheng et al., 1997; Cohen et al., 1993; Ehrhardt et al., 1995; Harris et al., 1993; Jose et al., 1993; Mays et al., 1996; Ross et al., 1992; Weiss, 1993; Williams et al., 1996; Young et al., 1992).

---

[20]The term "women who have sex with women" is used in this section for several reasons: it captures women who have sex with women but do not otherwise identify as lesbian or feel attraction to women, a group that may possibly be more highly represented among injection drug users, and it allows consideration of whether female-to-female transmission of HIV occurs.

HIV-related research on WSW, regardless of sexual orientation, has been scarce yet notable for its unexpected findings:

- higher HIV seroprevalence rates among women who have sex with both women and men (i.e., behaviorally bisexual women) compared to their exclusively homosexual or heterosexual counterparts;
- high levels of risk for HIV infection through unprotected sex with men and through injection drug use; and
- risk for HIV infection of unknown magnitude owing to unprotected sex with women and artificial insemination with unscreened semen.

Although estimates vary, numerous studies have reported HIV positivity among WSW. A study conducted in San Francisco reported a 1% HIV seroprevalence rate in a sample of 498 self-identified lesbian and bisexual women, higher than that reported for childbearing women in California (0.2%) or for women sampled from a San Francisco population-based household survey (0.4%) (Lemp et al., 1995). Behaviorally bisexual women from a predominantly African-American STD clinic population in New York City were reported to have an 18% HIV seroprevalence rate compared to 11% among exclusively heterosexual women (Bevier et al., 1995). Also, a study of injection drug-using women in drug treatment in King County, Washington, reported that women who identified as lesbian or bisexual had 8% HIV seroprevalence rates compared to 1.5% among heterosexual women (Harris et al., 1993). Several other studies corroborate the findings that WSW, specifically behaviorally bisexual and drug-injecting WSW, seem to have higher HIV seroprevalence rates than exclusively heterosexual women (Cheng et al., 1997; Cohen et al., 1993; Ehrhardt et al., 1995; Jose et al., 1993; Ross et al., 1992; Weiss, 1993; Williams et al., 1996; Young et al., 1992).

Because WSW have been ignored in most HIV prevention efforts they may perceive their risk of HIV exposure to be lower than it actually is. In a survey of 1,086 WSW, risk perception for HIV acquisition was not as high as would have been expected given the proportion of risk behaviors reported: only 43% of the women with a history of a clear HIV risk factor perceived themselves to be at risk for HIV infection (Einhorn and

Polgar, 1994). The perception of little or no risk for HIV infection among WSW reflects continued misconceptions by medical providers and researchers about the sexual behaviors and potential drug use of WSW and may contribute to delays in the diagnosis of HIV-related symptoms and an underestimation of risk of HIV infection among these women.

The explanation for increased HIV seroprevalence rates among certain subgroups of WSW remains uncertain. Some researchers suggest it could be related to the reason (e.g., sensation seeking) that those WSW engage in behaviors that increase HIV risk (Kalichman and Rompa, 1995); substance abuse (Solomon et al., 1996); sexual identity confusion (Gómez et al., 1996); or childhood sexual abuse (Widom and Kuhns, 1996). Other explanations are more closely linked to the fact that some WSW may be more likely to have sex or share needles with men who have sex with men or to be part of other social networks with high HIV seroprevalence rates (Deren et al., 1996; Turner et al., 1998).

Possible Sources of HIV Infection Among Women Who Have Sex with Women. Although WSW can be found in the same HIV exposure categories as women in general, including injection drug use, heterosexual contact, history of blood transfusions, and "no identified risk" (Chu et al., 1990; Kennedy et al., 1995), the precise number in each category is unknown, in part because same-sex contact among women is not consistently reported on AIDS case report forms (Doll et al., in press). Nonetheless, unprotected sex with men and sharing of drug injection equipment are believed to account for most cases of HIV infection in WSW, just as they do for women in general. However, the range of sexual and drug-using practices among WSW still remains largely unknown.

Injection Drug Use. A significant risk factor for HIV infection is injection drug use. Female injection drug users (IDUs) who have sex with both women and men (i.e., are behaviorally bisexual) have higher levels of HIV infection and HIV-related risk behaviors than other injectors. The only other major subgroup of injectors consistently reported to have HIV infection rates as high or higher than behaviorally bisexual women are men who have sex with men. This increase in HIV infection and risk is not related in a simple and direct way to women IDUs' sexual behaviors with other women. Thus, the patterns of HIV transmission cannot be accounted for by female-to-female transmission. Nor does HIV infection appear to be accounted for by any increased involvement in prostitution. Some differences in risk, however, may be accounted for by differences in risk networks. For example, women IDUs who have sex with women may be more likely to share needles or have sex with gay men, a particularly high-risk group for HIV infection.

Having Male Sexual Partners. Heterosexual activity among WSW presents a further avenue for entry of HIV into this population. The National Lesbian and Bisexual Women's Health Survey reported that 16% of 6,146 respondents were currently having sex with both male and female partners and that many women reported contracting an STD from a female partner, including 135 with herpes, 102 with chlamydia, 100 with genital warts, 16 with gonorrhea, 9 with hepatitis, and 1 with HIV (Cochran et al., 1996; Gage, 1994). Researchers at the University of Washington analyzed client records from the Harborview STD Clinic in Seattle from 1993 through 1995 to determine the characteristics of WSW seeking care at the clinic. Among all women who reported sex with men (12,307 women; 99% of all subjects), a report of having had sex with women in the prior two months was associated with significantly higher prevalence of HIV-related risk behaviors (Marrazzo et al., 1996b). Finally, female adolescents who have sex with other females are especially likely to engage in unprotected sex with both male and female partners (Hunter et al., 1993). Several other studies on sexual behaviors in WSW have reported a significant percentage (80 to 98%) of women who both identified themselves as lesbian and had engaged in heterosexual intercourse in their lifetime. Of particular concern regarding HIV transmission was the finding across several studies that a significant percentage of women (16 to 34%) reported having had sex with men who had sex with men (Cochran et al., 1996; Gómez et al., 1996; Lemp et al., 1995; Reinisch et al., 1990; Ziemba-Davis et al., 1996). Other research on heterosexual behaviors in lesbians has reported that as many as 21% of subjects reported anal intercourse during sexual activity with a man (Bell and Weinberg, 1978). These patterns of heterosexual behavior may put WSW at increased risk for HIV infection.

Female-to-Female Transmission of HIV. Research on female-to-female transmission of HIV has been virtually absent and continues to constitute a gap in the scientific literature on HIV transmission. The only study to date of HIV–serodiscordant lesbian couples (i.e., where one partner is HIV positive and the other HIV negative) was conducted in Italy and found that among the 18 lesbian couples participating in the study there were significant rates of high-risk sexual activities, but there was no evidence of female-to-female transmission of HIV (Raiteri et al., 1994a). Although the validity of these findings has been questioned owing to the small sample size and limited follow-up, they are consistent with the small number of identified cases of potential female-to-female transmission in the United States (Marmor et al., 1986; Monzon and Capellan, 1987; Perry et al., 1989). More systematic attempts to identify cases of female-to-female transmission of HIV are currently underway by the CDC (CDC, 1996). The lack of information about female-to-female transmission of HIV is particularly problematic for serodiscordant couples. Understanding the relationship of self-defined sexual identity, sexual behaviors, and risk of HIV infection is critical for all populations of WSW.

Substance Use Among Lesbians

In the 1996 National Household Survey on Drug Abuse (SAMHSA, 1997) 4.2% of women surveyed reported some illicit drug use during the past month (e.g., marijuana, cocaine, hallucinogens, heroin). About 10% of 15- to 44-year-old pregnant women and women with children in the household reported illicit drug use during the previous year; about 19% of women with no children reported such use. Slightly more than 40% of women aged 15 to 44 reported some previous use of illicit drugs during their lifetime. Alcohol use in the past month was reported by 43.6% of women surveyed; 8.7% reported binge alcohol use, and 1.9% reported heavy alcohol use.

Use of Alcohol Among Lesbians. [21] Data on the use of alcohol among lesbians are not available from population-based samples or large-

---

[21]This section is based largely on the workshop presentation made by Dr. Tonda Hughes.

scale epidemiological studies focusing on alcohol use, although this area has received some research attention. Nonetheless, reviews of lesbian health research consistently include alcohol abuse as a problem for which lesbians appear to be at greater risk than heterosexual women (Cassidy and Hughes, 1997; Eliason, 1996; Haas, 1994; O'Hanlan, 1995; Rosser, 1993; Skinner and Otis, 1996), and alcohol abuse has been widely viewed as a prevalent and serious problem among lesbians (Cabaj, 1992, 1996; Finnegan and McNally, 1990; Glaus, 1989; Hall, 1993; NGLTF, 1993; Skinner, 1994).

Data across a wide range of non-probability small-sample studies suggest that about 30% of lesbians may have alcohol problems (Bloomfield, 1993; Hall, 1993). However, this estimate may be inflated since these studies have generally had a number of methodological problems, including the fact that subjects have often been recruited using convenience sampling from settings in which alcohol consumption is likely to occur (e.g., bars). Further, it has been suggested that contemporary patterns of alcohol use among lesbians may be lower because bars have become a less important component of the lesbian culture as other options for social gathering have become increasingly available (Hall, 1993).

Despite methodological limitations of the research on alcohol use among lesbians (e.g., the use of samples from bars or other settings likely to attract people who consume higher levels of alcohol), some tentative patterns emerge across studies:

- A smaller percentage of lesbians compared to heterosexual women abstains from alcohol. Even when rates of heavy drinking among lesbians and heterosexual women are found to be reasonably comparable, rates of reported alcohol problems are higher in lesbians than in heterosexual women.
- Relationships among some demographic characteristics and drinking behaviors differ for lesbians and heterosexual women, particularly for age-related drinking patterns.
- A greater percentage of lesbians than heterosexual women describe themselves as being in recovery from alcohol abuse or alcoholism.

Lesbians have the same risk factors for alcohol abuse as other women do, including stress, anxiety, depression, genetic predisposition, and histories of childhood sexual abuse or violence. Some possible reasons for increased alcohol use among lesbians have been speculated; however, as with most research on lesbian health, these hypotheses should be considered tentative, particularly given the lack of attention to issues of social class in much of the existing research, including the following findings from Hughes and Wilsnack (1997):

• **Fewer roles, responsibilities, and social norms that limit drinking.** Although increasing numbers of lesbians are having children and many are in long-term committed relationships, lesbians are still less likely than heterosexual women to have children and to engage in other social and family roles that serve to limit drinking among heterosexual women. In addition, although this too is changing, there are fewer social norms against drinking in some lesbian communities and lesbians in general are likely less constrained by traditional gender role norms for women that serve to limit drinking.

• **Partner's drinking.** Women in general tend to drink like their intimate partners and lesbians are likely no exception. In addition, because lesbian relationships may tend to be characterized by greater intimacy and shared activities than heterosexual relationships, problem drinking of partners may have an even greater impact on lesbians' drinking.

Large-scale studies using probability sampling methods and appropriate non-lesbian comparison groups are needed to better assess and understand the patterns of alcohol use among lesbians.

Use of Illegal Drugs. Very few data are available to document the use of illegal drugs by lesbians. Skinner and Otis (1996) compared data on substance use from a multiple-recruitment source convenience sample of lesbians from two southern metropolitan areas with population-based survey data from similar geographical areas. They found that lesbians reported greater use of cigarettes, marijuana, inhalants, and cocaine than did women in general (Skinner and Otis, 1996). In the NLHCS, 47% of those surveyed reported some marijuana use (14% reporting at least weekly use),

19% reported some cocaine use, and about 1% reported ever using heroin (Bradford et al., 1994b).

Injection Drug Use Among Women Who Have Sex with Women. IDUs are a subgroup of drug users of particular interest because this practice significantly increases risk for transmission of HIV and hepatitis B and C and for other health problems. According to the 1996 National Household Survey on Drug Abuse (NHSDA; SAMHSA, 1997), in the past year less than one-half of 1% of women in general reported using heroin, the illicit drug most often associated with injection drug use.[22] It is not known, however, what proportion of these women administered heroin intravenously versus some other means of administration. Nor is it known what percentage of these women are WSW or women who identify as lesbian because probability-based data are not available on the percentage of lesbians who are IDUs. Nonetheless, several studies targeting self-identified lesbians and bisexual women have reported that between 2 and 6% of the women in their samples were injection drug users (Gómez et al., 1996; Lemp et al., 1995; Stevens, 1993).

A number of studies targeting female injection drug users have looked at the percentage of women in their samples who identify as lesbian or bisexual or who report having sex with other women (Friedman, 1998). Research questions about WSW were not the primary purpose of these drug use studies and drug-using women were recruited without regard to sexual orientation. Although data from these studies do not tell us what percentage of WSW are also IDUs, they are useful for establishing the fact that injection drug use is a problem that exists for these women just as it exists to some degree for women in general. They may also be useful for exploring whether lesbians or WSW are disproportionally represented among IDUs and thus would be at risk for the consequences of injection drug use.

A significant number of studies of female IDUs have reported WSW in their cohorts (Cheng et al., 1997; Harris et al., 1993; Jose et al., 1993;

---

[22]These figures likely represent an underestimation of the actual level of heroin use in the population, because the NHSDA captures only a small number of heavy drug users, and those who use heroin may fail to disclose this information (SAMHSA, 1997). Nonetheless, the data clearly show that heroin use is a rare behavior among women in general.

Ross et al., 1992; Weissman, 1990). In samples from a variety of settings (e.g., drug abuse treatment programs, street settings, and jails), findings suggest that the proportion of WSW among drug-injecting women may be higher than the proportion of WSW in the U.S. population as a whole. However, reported figures vary widely, in part because studies have sampled different populations and in part because they have used different measures to assess sexual orientation. For example, in a study of 6,667 women injection drug users participating in a multisite national study of IDUs and crack users, 12.5% reported that they identified as lesbian or bisexual or indicated that they had engaged in same-sex behavior during the past 30 days (Deren et al., 1996). In another study, which compared sexual risk behaviors of 39 HIV-positive and 37 HIV-negative inner-city women with a history of injection drug use, 28% reported being lesbian and 48% reported having had sex with a woman at least once in their lives (Ehrhardt et al., 1995).

By way of comparison, in the NHSLS,[23] 2.6% of women living in the 12 largest central cities reported having a lesbian or bisexual identity, and 6.5% reported that they had ever had sex with another woman (Laumann et al., 1994). These estimates are not, however, based on samples that more closely reflect the populations from whom studies of drug injectors primarily recruit their samples (e.g., working class or poor women, those from racial or ethnic minority backgrounds), so extreme caution should be used in making comparisons. These data on same-sex sexual behavior among IDUs, moreover, can easily be misinterpreted. That same-sex sexual behavior appears to occur at higher frequency among female IDUs than it does among similar non-injection drug-using women does not necessarily mean that lesbians are at higher risk of being IDUs. Data are not yet available, however, to determine the risk for lesbians.

It is important to consider that the proportion of lesbians, bisexuals, or WSW who are willing to disclose their sexual orientation or same-sex sexual behavior may be considerably higher among IDUs than among those who either are not drug injectors or are unwilling to disclose their drug use behavior. It is also important to note that for some women

---

[23]The NHSLS surveyed nearly 3,500 adults between the ages of 18 and 59, living in the United States, about their sexual practices (Laumann et al., 1994). The study was conducted by the National Opinion Research Center and supported by private funds.

IDUs, having sex with other women is a situational behavior (e.g., having sex in exchange for drugs or shelter or having sex while incarcerated). Such instances of sexual practice may not accurately reflect their sexual identity or desires. In the NHSLS, only 13% of the women who reported any adult same-gender sexuality engaged in same-sex sexual behavior without also having same-sex desires or a lesbian identity (Laumann et al., 1994). It is unknown, however, what percentage of female IDUs fall into this category.

SUGGESTED AREAS FOR RESEARCH

The committee believes that the following dimensions should be considered when determining the priority of lesbian health research areas: burden of disease, public health risk, theoretical underpinnings, and presence of conflicting findings in areas with significant clinical consequences.

The committee concludes that there are significant gaps in what is known about lesbian health with respect to numerous health conditions, including possible risk and protective factors. In addition, there are significant gaps in what is known about the health of lesbians across the life span and about their access to health services. Further, the committee concludes that it is particularly important that research on lesbian health issues consider how health problems vary along dimensions of race and ethnicity, social class, geographic region, and birth cohort (or age). Both qualitative and quantitative studies, as well as longitudinal studies, are needed.

The committee has identified a number of suggested areas for research on lesbian health, which are presented in Box 2.2. This list is not intended to be exhaustive nor does it set absolute priorities for research. Rather, it illustrates the range of issues in need of attention. The committee strongly believes that in all of these areas studies should be conducted to increase understanding of the health of lesbians of all social classes and racial and ethnic groups.

BOX 2.2
Suggested Areas for Further Research on Lesbian Health

General Risk and Protective Factors

- Risk and protective factors across the life span; coping and resiliency factors
- Impact of homophobia, prejudice, and discrimination on physical and mental health
- Dietary patterns of lesbians and prevalence of overweight and other eating disorders
- Childbearing patterns of lesbians
- Use of oral contraceptives among lesbians
- Involvement of lesbians in lesbian-centered community organizations and activities and their impact on lesbian health
- Lesbian social support networks
- Sources of stress for lesbians, and the impact of stress on their physical and mental health

Life-Span Development

- Interventions specifically geared to prevent health risk behaviors and events among lesbian adolescents (e.g., STDs, cigarette smoking, substance abuse)
- Process of coming out and what constitutes a psychologically healthy coming out
- Factors that help or hinder development of healthy self-esteem in lesbian adolescents
- Development of lesbian sexual identity
- Specific physical and mental health concerns of lesbians as they age, from childhood to old age
- Career patterns and workplace experiences

Mental Health

- Prevalence of mental disorders among lesbians, including major depression
- Relationships between lesbians and their family members and their influences on mental health
- Development of sexual orientation
- Impact of multiple minority statuses (e.g., being lesbian and a member of a racial or ethnic minority group) on the formation of lesbian identity and on mental health
- Normative mental health for lesbians across the life span
- Relationship between suicide and sexual orientation, particularly during adolescence
- Effectiveness of various therapeutic approaches with lesbians

Continued

BOX 2.2 *Continued*

- Lesbian motherhood, including studies of children born into or adopted by lesbian-parented families
  - Utilization of mental health services
  - Stress effects of various aspects of homophobia and their influence on health
    - Impact of violence and other hate crimes on the lives of lesbians
    - History of having experienced childhood sexual abuse

Cancer

- Population-based studies to determine the incidence of cancer among lesbians
  - Prevalence of cancer risk factors among lesbians
  - Frequency of Pap tests among lesbians
  - Patterns of preventive behaviors among lesbians (e.g., mammograms, Pap tests)

Cardiovascular Diseases

- Population-based studies to determine incidence of cardiovascular diseases among lesbians
  - Prevalence of risk factors for cardiovascular diseases among lesbians

HIV/AIDS

- Mechanisms operating to increase HIV risk among injection drug-using WSW
  - Research on the risk networks of injection drug-using WSW
  - High-risk sexual and injection behaviors among WSW
  - Risks of transmission through specific female-to-female sex behaviors

Sexually Transmitted Diseases

- Risks of STD (including HIV) transmission through female-to-female sex
  - Measurements of sexual partnerships and sexual networks (including HIV status of male sex partners)
  - Prevalence of bacterial vaginosis among women who have sex with women
  - Sexual histories of lesbians, including history of sexual contact with men

Substance Abuse

- Etiology of substance use and abuse (including alcohol) among lesbians
  - Drug-using patterns among lesbians
  - Extent to which treatment facilities for alcohol and drug problems provide adequate care for lesbian clients

---

BOX 2.2 *Continued*

- Prevalence of cigarette smoking among lesbians and patterns of tobacco use
- Prevalence of heavy drug use and injection drug use among lesbians
- Prevalence of infections related to injection drug use, such as hepatitis B and C
- Associations between childhood sexual abuse and substance abuse, including alcohol abuse

Service Delivery and Access to Services

- Lesbians' patterns of use of health care services
- Models of care that act to remove barriers of access to care for lesbians
- Impact of managed care on quality of care for lesbians
- What constitutes a basic standard of care for lesbian health
- Whether cultural competency training of providers on the needs of lesbians will increase sensitive delivery of health care for lesbians
- Access to health insurance for lesbians
- Need for prevention and treatment intervention models targeted specifically toward lesbians
- Barriers to care for lesbians, including adolescent lesbians

---

REFERENCES

Adler NE, Boyce WT, Chesney MA, Folkman S, Syme SL. 1993. Socioeconomic inequalities in health. *Journal of the American Medical Association* 269(24):3140–3145.

Adler NE, Boyce T, Chesney MA, Cohen S, Folkman S, Kahn RL, Syme SL. 1994. Socioeconomic status and health: The challenge of the gradient. *American Psychologist* 49(1):15–24.

American Cancer Society. 1997. Cancer Facts and Figures—1997 [WWW Document]. URL www.cancer.org/statistics/97cff/ (accessed December 1 and 3, 1997).

Anderson RN, Kochanek KD, Murphy SL. 1997. Report of Final Mortality Statistics, 1995. *Monthly Vital Statistics Report 45(11, suppl. 2)*. DHHS Pub No. (PHS) 97-1120. Rockville, MD: National Center for Health Statistics.

APA (American Psychological Association). 1997.

Bell AP, Weinberg MS. *1978. Homosexualities: A Study of Diversity Among Men and Women*. New York: Simon and Schuster.

Berger BJ, Kolton S, Zenilman JM, Cummings MC, Feldman J, McCormack WM. 1995. Bacterial vaginosis in lesbians: A sexually transmitted disease. *Clinical Infectious Diseases* 21(6):1402–1405.

Bevier PJ, Chaisson MA, Heffernan RT, Castro KG. 1995. Women at a sexually transmitted disease clinic who reported same-sex contact: Their HIV seroprevalence and risk behaviors. *American Journal of Public Health* 85(10):1366–1371.

Biddle BS. 1993. *Health Status Indicators for Washington Area Lesbians and Bisexual Women: A Report on the Lesbian Health Clinic's First Year.* Washington, DC: Whitman-Walker Clinic.

Black J, Underwood J. 1998. Young, female, and gay: Lesbian students and the school environment. *Professional School Counseling* 1(3):15–20.

Bloomfield K. 1993. A comparison of alcohol consumption between lesbians and heterosexual women in an urban population. *Drug and Alcohol Dependence* 33:257–269.

Bowen D, Hickman KM, Powers D. 1997. Importance of psychological variables in understanding risk perceptions and breast cancer screening of African-American women. *Womens Health* 3(3–4):227–242.

Bradford J, Ryan C. 1988. *The National Lesbian Health Care Survey: Final Report.* Washington, DC: National Lesbian and Gay Health Foundation.

Bradford J, Plumb M, White J, Ryan C. 1994a. Information Transfer Strategies to Support Lesbian Research. *Psychological and Behavioral Factors in Women's Health: Creating an Agenda for the 21st Century—Conference Proceedings.* Washington, DC: American Psychological Association.

Bradford J, Ryan C, Rothblum ED. 1994b. National Lesbian Health Care Survey: Implications for mental health care. *Journal of Consulting and Clinical Psychology* 62(2):228–242.

Brewaeys A, van Ball EV. 1997. Lesbian motherhood: The impact on child development and family functioning. *Journal of Psychosomatic Obstetrics and Gynaecology* 18:116.

Brewaeys A, Devroey P, Helmerhorst FM, Van Hall EV, Ponjaert I. 1995. Lesbian mothers who conceived after donor insemination: A follow-up study. *Human Reproduction* 10(10):2731–2735.

Brewaeys A, Ponjaert I, van Ball EV, Golombok S. 1997. Donor insemination: Child development and family functioning in lesbian mother families. *Human Reproduction* 12:1349–1359.

Buhrke RA, Ben-Ezra LA, Hurley ME, Ruprecht LJ. 1992. Content analysis and methodological critique of articles concerning lesbian and gay male issues in counseling journals. *Journal of Counseling Psychology* 39(1):91–99.

Bybee D, Roeder V. 1990. *Michigan Lesbian Health Survey: Results Relevant to AIDS. A Report to the Michigan Organization for Human Rights and the Michigan Department of Public Health.* Lansing: Michigan Department of Health and Human Services.

Cabaj RP. 1992. Substance abuse in the gay and lesbian community. In: Lowenson J, Ruiz P, Millman R, eds. *Substance Abuse: A Comprehensive Textbook.* Baltimore, MD: Williams and Wilkins. Pp. 852–860.

Cabaj RP. 1996. Substance abuse in gay men, lesbians, and bisexuals. In: Cabaj RP, Stein TS, eds. *Textbook of Homosexuality and Mental Health.* Washington, DC: American Psychiatric Press, Inc. Pp. 783–799.

Cassidy MA, Hughes TL. 1997. Lesbian health: Barriers to care. In: McElmurry BJ, Parker RS, eds. *Annual Review of Women's Health,* Vol. 3. New York: National League for Nursing Press. Pp. 67–87.

CDC (Centers for Disease Control and Prevention). 1996. *Sexually Transmitted Disease Surveillance, 1995.* Atlanta, GA: Centers for Disease Control and Prevention, Division of STD Prevention.

CDC. 1997. *HIV/AIDS Surveillance Report, 1996.* Vol. 8 (No. 2). Atlanta, GA: Centers for Disease Control and Prevention.

Cheng FK, Ford WL, Weber MD, Cheng S-Y, Kerndt PR. 1997. A probability-based approach for predicting HIV infection in a low prevalent population of injection drug users. *AIDS Education and Prevention* 7:28–34.

Chu SY, Buehler JW, Fleming PL, Berkelman RL. 1990. Epidemiology of reported cases of AIDS in lesbians, United States 1980–89. *American Journal of Public Health* 80(11): 1380–1381.

Chu SY, Hammett TA, Buehler JW. 1992. Update: Epidemiology of reported cases of AIDS in women who report sex only with other women, United States, 1980–1991 [letter]. *AIDS* 6:518–519.

Cochran SD, Bybee D, Gage S, Mays VM. 1996. Prevalence of HIV-related self-reported sexual behaviors, sexually transmitted diseases, and problems with drugs and alcohol in 3 large surveys of lesbian and bisexual women: A look into a segment of the community. *Women's Health Research on Gender, Behavior, and Policy* 2(1–2):11–33.

Cochran SD, Mays VM. 1994. Depressive distress among homosexually active African-American men and women. *American Journal of Psychiatry* 151(4):524–529.

Cohen H, Marmor M, Wolfe H, Ribble D. 1993. Risk assessment of HIV transmission among lesbians [letter]. *Journal of Acquired Immune Deficiency Syndrome* 6(10):1173–1174.

D'Augelli AR, Hershberger SL. 1993. Lesbian, gay, and bisexual youth in community settings: Personal challenges and mental health problems. *American Journal of Community Psychology* 21(4):421–448.

Denenberg R. 1995. Report on lesbian health. *Women's Health Issues* 5(2):81–91.

Deren S, Goldstein M, Williams M, Stark M, Estrada A, Friedman SR, Young RM. 1996. Sexual orientation, HIV risk behavior, and serostatus in a multisite sample of drug-injecting and crack-using women. *Women's Health: Research on Gender, Behavior, and Policy* 2(1–2):35–47.

Edwards A, Thin RN. 1990. Sexually transmitted diseases in lesbians. *International Journal of STD and AIDS* 1:178–181.

Ehrhardt AA, Nostlinger C, Meyer-Bahlburg HFL, Exner TM, Gruen RS, Yingling SL, Gorman JM, El-Sadr W, Sorrell SJ. 1995. Sexual risk behavior among women with injection drug use histories. *Journal of Psychology and Human Sexuality* 7:99–119.

Einhorn L, Polgar M. 1994. HIV-risk behavior among lesbians and bisexual women. *AIDS Education and Prevention* 6(6):514–523.

Eliason MJ. 1996. Caring for the lesbian, gay, or bisexual patient: Issues for critical care nurses. *Critical Care Nursing Quarterly* 19(1):65–72.

Englert Y. 1994. Artificial insemination of single women and lesbian women with donor semen. Artificial insemination with donor semen: Particular requests. *Human Reproduction* 9(11):1969–1971.

Eschenbach DA. 1993. Bacterial vaginosis and anaerobes in obstetric–gynecologic infection. *Clinical Infectious Diseases* 16:S282–S287.

FBI (Federal Bureau of Investigation). 1996. *Uniform Crime Reports: Hate Crime Statistics 1996.* Clarksburg, WV: U.S. Department of Justice, Federal Bureau of Investigation.

Ferris DG, Batish S, Wright TC, Cushing C, Scott EH. 1996. A neglected lesbian health concern: Cervical neoplasia. *Journal of Family Practice* 43(6):581–584.

Finnegan DG, McNally EB. 1990. Lesbian women. In: Engs RC ed. *Women: Alcohol and Other Drugs.* Dubuque, IA: Kendall/Hunt Publishing Company. Pp. 149–156.

Fontaine JH, Hammond NL. 1996. Counseling issues with gay and lesbian adolescents. *Adolescence* 31(124):817–830.

Gage S. 1994. Preliminary findings: The National Lesbian and Bisexual Women's Health Survey. *Lesbian Health Project of Los Angeles.* New York: National Lesbian and Gay Health Conference.

Garnets L, Hancock KA, Cochran SD, Goodchilds J, Peplau LA. 1991. Issues in psychotherapy with lesbians and gay men. A survey of psychologists. *American Psychologist* 46(9):964–972.

Geddes VA. 1994. Lesbian expectations and experiences with family doctors. How much does the physician's sex matter to lesbians? *Canadian Family Physician* 40:908–920.

Glaus KO. 1989. Alcoholism, chemical dependency and the lesbian client. *Women and Therapy* 8(2):131–144.

Gold MA, Perrin EC, Futterman D, Friedman SB. 1994. Children of gay or lesbian parents. *Pediatrics in Review* 15(9):354–358.

Golombok S, Tasker F. 1994. Donor insemination for single heterosexual and lesbian women: Issues concerning the welfare of the child. *Human Reproduction* 9(11):1972–1976.

Gómez CA. 1994. Lesbians at risk for HIV: An unresolved debate. In: Greene B, Herek GM eds. *Psychosocial Perspectives on Lesbian and Gay Issues, Vol. I: Lesbian and Gay Psychology: Theory, Research, and Clinical Applications.* Thousand Oaks, CA: Sage.

Gómez CA, Garcia DR, Kegebein VJ, Shade SB, Hernandez SR. 1996. Sexual identity versus sexual behavior: Implications for HIV prevention strategies for women who have sex with women. *Women's Health: Research on Gender, Behavior, and Policy* 2(1–2):91–109.

Greene B. 1994a. Ethnic-minority lesbians and gay men: Mental health and treatment issues. *Journal of Consulting and Clinical Psychology* 62(2):243–251.

Greene B. 1994b. Lesbian women of color: Triple jeopardy. In: Comas-Díaz L, Greene B, eds. *Women of Color: Integrating Ethnic and Gender Identities in Psychotherapy.* New York: Guilford Press. Pp. 389–427.

Greene B, Boyd-Franklin N. 1996. African American lesbians: Issues in couples therapy. In: Laird J, Green RJ, eds. *Lesbians and Gays in Couples and Families: A Handbook for Therapists.* San Francisco, CA: Jossey-Bass. Pp. 251–271.

Haas AP. 1994. Lesbian health issues: An overview. In: Dan AJ, ed. *Reframing Women's Health: Multidisciplinary Research and Practice.* Thousand Oaks, CA: Sage Publications. Pp. 339–356.

Hall JM. 1993. Lesbians and alcohol: Patterns and paradoxes in medical notions and lesbians' beliefs. *Journal of Psychoactive Drugs* 25(2):109–119.

Harris NV, Thiede H, McGough JP, Gordon D. 1993. Risk factors for HIV infection among injection drug users: Results of blinded surveys in drug treatment centers, King County, Washington 1988–1991. *Journal of Acquired Immune Deficiency Syndrome* 6(11):1275–1282.

Hillier SL, Nugent RP, Eschenbach DA, Krohn MA, Gibbs RS, Martin DH, Cotch MF, Edelman R, Pastorek JG, Rao AV, McNellis D, Regan JA, Carey JC, Klebanoff MA. 1995. Association between bacterial vaginosis and preterm delivery of a low-birth-weight infant. *New England Journal of Medicine* 333:1737–1742.

Hughes TL, Wilsnack SC. 1997. Use of alcohol among lesbians: Research and clinical implications. *American Journal of Orthopsychiatry* 67(1):20–36.

Hunter J, Rosario M. Rotheram-Borus MJ. 1993. Sexual and substance abuse acts that place adolescent lesbians at risk for HIV. In: *IXth International Conference on AIDS and the IVth STD World Congress*. Berlin: IXth International Conference on AIDS.

IOM (Institute of Medicine). 1993. *Access to Health Care in America*. Washington, DC: National Academy Press.

IOM. 1994. *Reducing Risks for Mental Disorders: Frontiers for Preventive Intervention Research*. Washington, DC: National Academy Press.

IOM. 1997. *The Hidden Epidemic: Confronting Sexually Transmitted Diseases*. Washington, DC: National Academy Press.

Jose B, Friedman SR, Neaigus A, Curtis R, Grund JPC, Goldstein M, Ward T, Des Jarlais DC. 1993. Syringe-mediated drug-sharing (backloading): A new risk factor for HIV among injecting drug users. *AIDS* 7:1653–1660.

Kalichman SC, Rompa D. 1995. Sexual sensation seeking and Sexual Compulsivity Scales: Reliability, validity, and predicting HIV risk behavior. *Journal of Personality Assessment* 65(3):586–601.

Kalton G. 1993. Sampling considerations in research on HIV risk and illness. In: Ostrow DG, Kessler RC, eds. *Methodological Issues in AIDS Behavioral Research*. New York: Plenum Press. Pp. 53–74.

Kawachi I, Kennedy BP. 1997. Health and social cohesion: Why care about income inequality? *British Medical Journal* 314:1037–1040.

Kennedy MB, Scarlett MI, Duerr AC, Chu SY. 1995. Assessing HIV risk among women who have sex with women: Scientific and communication issues. *Journal of the American Medical Womens' Association* 50(3–4):103–107.

Kessler RC, McGonagle KA, Zhao S, Nelson CB, Hughes M, Eshleman S, Wittchen H-U, Kendler KS. 1994. Lifetime and 12-month prevalance of DSM-III-R psychiatric disorders in the United States: Results from the National Comorbidity Survey. *Archives of General Psychiatry* 51:8–19.

Krieger N, Sidney S. 1996. Blood pressure: The CARDIA study of young black and white adults. *American Journal of Public Health* 86(10):1370–1378.

Krieger N, Sidney S. 1997. Prevalence and health implications of anti-gay discrimination: A study of black and white women and men in the CARDIA cohort. *International Journal of Health Services* 27(1):157–176.

Kripke CC, Vaias L, Elliott A. 1994. The importance of taking a sensitive sexual history. *Journal of the American Medical Association* 271(9):713.

Laumann EO, Gagnon JH, Michael RT, Michaels S. 1994. *The Social Organization of Sexuality: Sexual Practices in the United States*. Chicago: University of Chicago Press.

Lechner ME, Vogel ME, Garcia-Shelton LM, Leichter JL, Steibel KR. 1993. Self-reported medical problems of adult female survivors of childhood sexual abuse. *Journal of Family Practice* 36(6):633–638.

Lemp GF, Jones M, Kellogg TA, Nieri GN, et al. 1995. HIV seroprevalence and risk behaviors among lesbians and bisexual women in San Francisco and Berkeley, California. *American Journal of Public Health* 85(11):1549–1552.

Liu P, Chan CS. 1996. Lesbian, gay, and bisexual Asian Americans and their families. In: Laird J, Green R-J, eds. *Lesbians and Gays in Couples and Families: A Handbook for Therapists*. San Francisco: Jossey-Bass. Pp. 137–152.

Lynch MA. 1993. When the patient is also a lesbian. *AWHONNS Clinical Issues in Perinatal Womens Health Nursing* 4(2):196–202.

Marmor M, Weiss LR, Lyden M. Weiss SH, Saxinger WC, Spira TJ, Feorino PM. *Annals of Internal Medicine* 105(6):969.

Marrazzo JM, Koutsky LA, Stine K, Kuypers JM, Grubert TA, Galloway DA, Kiviat NB, Handsfield HH. In press. Genital human papillomavirus infection in women who have sex with women. *Journal of Infectious Diseases*.

Marrazzo JM, Stine K, Handsfield HH, Kiviat NB, Koutsky LA. 1996a. Epidemiology of sexually transmitted diseases and cervical neoplasia in lesbian and bisexual women. *18th Conference of the National Lesbian and Gay Health Association*, Seattle, WA, July 13–16.

Marrazzo JM, Stine K, Handsfield HH, Kiviat NB, Koutsky LA. 1996b. HIV-related risk behavior in a community-based sample of women who have sex with women. *XI International Conference on AIDS/HIV*, Vancouver, Canada, July 7–12.

Mays VM. 1996. Are lesbians at risk for HIV infection? *Women's Health: Research on Gender, Behavior, and Policy* 2(1–2):1–9.

Mays VM, Cochran SD, Pies C, Chu SY, Ehrhardt AA. 1996. The risk of HIV infection for lesbians and other women who have sex with women: Implications for HIV research, prevention, policy, and services. *Women's Health: Research on Gender, Behavior, and Policy* 2(1–2):119–139.

McEwen BS. 1998. Protective and damaging effects of stress mediators. *Seminars in Medicine of the Beth Israel Deaconess Medical Center* 338(3):171–179.

Merrill JM, Laux LF, Thornby JI. 1990. Why doctors have difficulty with sex histories. *Southern Medical Journal* 83(6):613–617.

Monzon OT, Capellan JM. 1987. Female-to-female transmission of HIV. *Lancet* 2(8549):40–41.

Moran N. 1996. Lesbian health care needs. *Canadian Family Physician* 42:879–884.

Morrow DF. 1993. Social work with gay and lesbian adolescents [published erratum appears in *Social Work* 1994 39(2):166]. *Social Work* 38(6):655–660.

Muehrer P. 1995. Suicide and sexual orientation: A critical summary of recent research and directions for future research. *Suicide and Life-Threatening Behavior* 25(Suppl):72–81.

NCI (National Cancer Institute). 1997. Cancer Facts 5.6: Lifetime Probability of Breast Cancer in American Women [WWW Document]. URL rex.nci.nih.gov/INFO_CANCER/Cancer_facts/Section5/FS5_6.html (accessed December 1, 1997).

Neisen JH, Sandall H. 1990. Alcohol and other drug abuse in gay/lesbian populations: Related to victimization? *Journal of Psychology and Human Sexuality* 3(1):151–168.

NGLTF (National Gay and Lesbian Task Force). 1993. *Lesbian Health Issues and Recommendations*. Washington, DC: National Gay and Lesbian Task Force.

NGLTF. 1998. Capital Gains and Losses '97: A State by State Review of All Gay, Lesbian, Bisexual and Transgender Legislation in 1997. Review by Issue [WWW Document]. URL http://www.ngltf.org/97cgal/review.html (accessed February 12, 1998).

NHLBI (National Heart Lung and Blood Institute). 1997. Facts About Heart Disease and Women: Are You at Risk? [Updated August 1996] [WWW Document]. URL gopher://fido.nhlbi.nih.gov:70/00/...ealth/cardio/other/gp/hdwmnrsk.txt (accessed December 1, 1997).

O'Hanlan KA. 1995. Lesbian health and homophobia: Perspectives for the treating obstetrician/gynecologist. *Current Problems in Obstetrics, Gynecology and Fertility* 18(4):93–136.

O'Hanlan KA, Crum CP. 1996. Human papillomavirus-associated cervical intraepithelial neoplasia following lesbian sex. *Obstetrics and Gynecology* 4(Part 2):702–703.

Pattatucci AM, Hamer DH. 1995. Development and familiality of sexual orientation in females. *Behavior Genetics* 25(5):407–420.

Patterson CJ. 1992. Children of lesbian and gay parents. *Child Development* 63:1025–1042.

Patterson CJ. 1998. Sexual Orientation and Fertility. *Infertility in the Modern World. A Conference of the Cambridge Biosocial Society*. Cambridge, England, May 8, Cambridge, England: Cambridge Biosocial Society.

Perrin EC. 1996. Pediatricians and gay and lesbian youth. *Pediatrics in Review* 17(9):311–318.

Perry S, Jacobsberg L, Fogel K. 1989. Orogenital transmission of human immuno-deficiency virus. *Annals of Internal Medicine* 111(11):951–952.

Peters DK, Cantrell PJ. 1991. Factors distinguishing samples of lesbians and heterosexual women. *Journal of Homosexuality* 21:1–15.

Powch IG, Houston BK. 1996. Hostility, anger-in, and cardiovascular reactivity in white women. *Health Psychology* 15(3):200–208.

Price JH, Easton AN, Telljohann SK, Wallace PB. 1996. Perceptions of cervical cancer and Pap smear screening behavior by women's sexual orientation. *Journal of Community Health* 21(2):89–105.

Proctor CD, Groze VK. 1994. Risk factors for suicide among gay, lesbian, and bisexual youths. *Social Work* 39(5):504–513.

Raiteri R, Fora R, Sinicco A. 1994a. No HIV-1 transmission through lesbian sex. *Lancet* 344(8917):270.

Raiteri R, Fora R, Gioannini P, Russo R, Lucchini A, Terzi MG, Giacobbi D, Sinicco A. 1994b. Seroprevalence, risk factors and attitude to HIV-1 in a representative sample of lesbians in Turin. *Genitourinary Medicine* 70(3):200–205.

Rankow EJ. 1995a. Breast and cervical cancer among lesbians. *Women's Health Issues* 5(3):123–129.

Rankow EJ. 1995b. Lesbian health issues for the primary care provider. *Journal of Family Practice* 40(5):486–496. Comment in 41(3)224; discussion 227.

Reinisch JM, Ziemba-Davis M, Sanders SA. 1990. Sexual behavior and AIDS: Lessons from art and sex research. In: Voeller B, Reinisch JM, Gottlieb M eds. *AIDS and Sex: An Integrated Biomedical and Biobehavioral Approach*. New York: Oxford University Press. Pp. 37–80.

Remafedi G, French S, Story M, Resnick MD, Blum R. 1998. The relationship between suicide risk and sexual orientation: Results of a population-based study. *American Journal of Public Health* 88(1):57–60.

Reynolds G. 1994. HIV and lesbian sex. *Lancet* 344(8921):544–545.

Robb N. 1999. Medical schools seek to overcome "invisibility" of gay patients, gay issues in curriculum. *Canadian Medical Association Journal* 155(6):765–770. Comments in 155(6):709–711 and 155(12):1664.

Roberts SJ, Sorensen L. 1995. Lesbian health care: A review and recommendations for health promotion in primary care settings. *Nurse Practitioner* 20(6):42–47.

Robertson P, Schachter J. 1981. Failure to identify venereal disease in a lesbian population. *Sexually Transmitted Diseases* 8(2):75–76.

Robinson G, Cohen M. 1996. Gay, lesbian and bisexual health care issues and medical curricula. *Canadian Medical Association Journal* 155(6):709–711. Comments in 155(6):765–770 and 155(12):666.

Rohsenow DJ, Corbett R, Devine D. 1988. Molested as children: A hidden contribution to substance abuse? *Journal of Substance Abuse Treatment* 5:13–18.

Ross MW, Wodak A, Gold J, Miller ME. 1992. Differences across sexual orientation on HIV risk behaviors in injection drug users. *AIDS Care* 4(2):139–148.

Rosser S. 1993. Ignored, overlooked, or subsumed: Research on lesbian health and health care. *National Women's Studies Association Journal* 5(2):183–203.

Rothblum ED. 1994. "I only read about myself on bathroom walls": The need for research on the mental health of lesbians and gay men. *Journal of Consulting and Clinical Psychology* 62(2):213–220.

Russell JM, Azadian BS, Roberts AP, Talboys CA. 1995. Pharyngeal flora in a sexually active population. *International Journal of STD and AIDS* 6(3):211–215.

Ryan C, Futterman D, eds. 1997. *Adolescent Medicine: State of the Art Reviews. Special Issue on Lesbian and Gay Youth: Care and Counseling*. (8)2. Philadelphia: Hanley and Belfus, Inc.

SAMHSA (Substance Abuse and Mental Health Services Administration). 1997. *Preliminary Results from the 1996 National Household Survey on Drug Abuse*. DHHS Pub. No. (SMA) 97-3149. Rockville, MD: Substance Abuse and Mental Health Services Administration.

Savin-Williams RC. 1994. Verbal and physical abuse as stressors in the lives of lesbian, gay male, and bisexual youths: Associations with school problems, running away, substance abuse, prostitution, and suicide. Special Section: Mental health of lesbians and gay men. *Journal of Consulting and Clinical Psychology* 62(2):261–269.

Savin-Williams RC. 1996. Self-labeling and disclosure among gay, lesbian, and bisexual youths. In: Laird J, Green RJ eds. *Lesbians and Gays in Couples and Families: A Handbook for Therapists*. San Francisco, CA: Jossey-Bass. Pp. 153–182.

Savin-Williams RC, Rodriguez RG. 1993. A developmental, clinical perspective on lesbian, gay male, and bisexual youths. In: Gullotta TP, Adams GR, Montemayor R eds. *Adolescent Sexuality. Advances in Adolescent Development*. Newbury Park, CA: Sage Publications. Pp. 77–101.

Seeman TE, McEwen B. 1996. Impact of social environment characteristics on neuroendocrine regulation. *Psychosomatic Medicine* 58:459–471.

Skinner CJ, Stokes J, Kirlew Y, Kavanagh J, Forster GE. 1996. A case-controlled study of the sexual health needs of lesbians. *Genitourinary Medicine* 72(4):277–280.

Skinner WF. 1994. The prevalence and demographic predictors of illicit and licit drug use among lesbians and gay men. *American Journal of Public Health* 84(8):1307–1310.

Skinner WF, Otis MD. 1996. Drug and alcohol use among lesbian and gay people in a southern U.S. sample: Epidemiological, comparative, and methodological findings from the Triology Project. *Journal of Homosexuality* 30(3):59–92.

Skinner CJ, Stokes J, Kirlew Y, Kavanagh J, Forster GE. 1996. A case-controlled study of the sexual health needs of lesbians. *Genitourinary Medicine* 72(4):277–280.

Smith EM, Johnson SR, Guenther SM. 1985. Health care attitudes and experiences during gynecologic care among lesbians and bisexuals. *American Journal of Public Health* 75(9): 1085–1087.

Solomon L, Moore J, Gleghorn A, Astemborski J, Vlahov D. 1996. HIV testing behaviors in a population of inner-city women at high risk for HIV infection. *Journal of Acquired Immune Deficiency Syndrome and Human Retrovirology* 13(3):267–272.

Stevens PE. 1992. Lesbian health care research: A review of the literature from 1970 to 1990. *Health Care for Women International* 13(2):91–120.

Stevens PE. 1993. Lesbians and HIV: Clinical, research, and policy issues. *American Journal of Orthopsychiatry* 63(2):289–294.

Stevens PE. 1995. Structural and interpersonal impact of heterosexual assumptions on lesbian health care clients. *Nursing Research* 44(1):25–30.

Sullivan TR. 1994. Obstacles to effective child welfare service with gay and lesbian youths. *Child Welfare* 73(4):291–304.

Tasker F, Golombok S. 1995. Adults raised as children in lesbian families. *American Journal of Orthopsychiatry* 65(2):203–215.

Temple-Smith M, Hammond J, Pyett P, Presswell N. 1996. Barriers to sexual history taking in general practice. *Australian Family Physician* 25(9 Suppl. 2):673–679.

Tesar CM, Rovi SLD. 1998. Survey of curriculum on homosexuality/bisexuality in departments of family medicine. *Family Medicine* 30(4):283–287.

Trippet SE. 1994. Lesbians' mental health concerns. *Health Care for Women International* 15(4):317–323.

Troiden RR. 1988. Homosexual identity development. *Journal of Adolescent Health Care* 9:105–113.

Troiden RR. 1989. The formation of homosexual identities. *Journal of Homosexuality* 17:43–73.

Turner CF, Lessler JT, Devore J. 1992. Effects of mode administration and wording on reporting of drug use. In: Turner CF, Lessler JT, Gfroerer JD eds. *Survey Measurement of Drug Use: Methodological Issues.* DHHS Pub. No. 92-1929. Washington, DC: U.S. Government Printing Office.

Turner CF, Ku L, Rogers SM, Lindberg LD, Pleck JH, Sonenstein FL. 1998. Adolescent sexual behavior, drug use, and violence: Increased reporting with computer survey technology. *Science* 280:867–873.

Vollmer SA, Wells KB. 1989. The preparedness of freshman medical students for taking sexual histories. *Archives of Sexual Behavior* 18(2):167–177.

Waitkevicz J. 1997. Presentation at Institute of Medicine Committee on Lesbian Health Research Priorities, Washington, DC, October 6–7, 1997.

Weiss SH. 1993. Risk of HIV and other sexually transmitted diseases (STD) among (high risk bisexual and heterosexual) women in Northern New Jersey. Paper Presented at the IXth International Conference on AIDS. Berlin, June 1993.

Weissman G. 1990. Drug Use Patterns Among Gay and Bisexual Men and Lesbians in a National Study. Paper Presented at the National Gay and Lesbian Health Forum. July 19, 1990.

White JC. 1997. HIV risk assessment and prevention among lesbians and women who have sex with women: Practical information for clinicians. *Health Care for Women International* 18(2):1549–1552.

White JC, Dull VT. 1997. Health risk factors and health-seeking behavior in lesbians. *Journal of Women's Health* 6(1):103–112.

White J, Levinson W. 1993. Primary care of lesbian patients. *Journal of General Internal Medicine* 8(1):41–47.

White JC, Levinson W. 1995. Lesbian health care. What a primary care physician needs to know. *Western Journal of Medicine* 162(5):463–466.

Widom CS, Kuhns JB. 1996. Childhood victimization and subsequent risk for promiscuity, prostitution, and teenage pregnancy: A prospective study. *American Journal of Public Health* 86(11):1607–1612.

Williams ML, Elwood WN, Weatherby NL, Bowen AM, Zhao Z, Saunders LA, Montoya ID. 1996. An assessment of the risks of syphilis and HIV infection among a sample of not-in-treatment drug users in Houston, Texas. *AIDS Care* 8:671–682.

Wolfe A. 1998. *One Nation, After All: What Americans Really Think About God, Country, Family, Racism, Welfare, Immigration, Homosexuality, Work, the Right, the Left and Each Other.* New York: Viking Press.

Young RM, Weissman G, Cohen JB. 1992. Assessing the risk in the absence of information: HIV risk among women injection drug users who have sex with women. *AIDS and Public Policy Journal* 7:175–183.

Ziemba-Davis M, Sanders SA, Reinisch JM. 1996. Lesbians' sexual interactions with men: Behavioral bisexuality and risk for sexually transmitted disease (STD) and human immunodeficiency virus (HIV). *Women's Health: Research on Gender, Behavior, and Policy* 2(1–2):61–74.

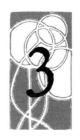

Methodological Challenges in Conducting Research on Lesbian Health

Conducting research on lesbian health presents numerous challenges because lesbians represent a subgroup of women for which standard definitions of the population are lacking and lesbians are not readily identifiable. These challenges are further compounded because many in the lesbian community distrust research and researchers and there has been little funding support for conducting research on lesbian health topics. It is not surprising, then, that methodologically rigorous large-scale studies are lacking in this area. Furthermore, a number of methodological challenges for comparing findings across studies are consistently found in lesbian health research.

1. Inconsistencies in the way sexual orientation is defined make it difficult to compare findings across studies. Studies have not been consistent in how they define a lesbian sexual orientation, with some focusing on sexual behavior and others focusing on identity or desire. Studies have also used a range of time frames in which to capture reports of past or present sexual behavior, some for example looking at behavior during the past six months or a year and others looking at lifetime behavior. As discussed in Chapter 1 these can all be appropriate ways of assessing sexual orientation depending on the needs of the study. However, researchers have usually failed to state how they define sexual orientation.

2. The lack of standard measures, including measures of sexual orientation, makes it difficult to compare findings across studies. Studies of lesbian health have lacked standard measures of sexual orientation including its three components—behavior, identity, and attraction or desire—which makes comparisons among studies difficult. In addition, like much other research on health–related behaviors, studies have often lacked standard measures of such variables as alcohol consumption and drinking behavior, depression, and childhood sexual abuse.

3. The use of small, nonprobability samples limits the generalizability of findings. Most lesbian health studies have relied on nonprobability samples. In particular, many studies have used convenience samples (e.g., from lesbian bars, music festivals, gay and lesbian organizations). As discussed later, these nonprobability samples are not likely to be representative of the population of lesbians. Further, most lesbian women sampled have been white, middle-class, well educated, and between 25 and 40 years old (Hughes and Wilsnack, 1997) and thus may not be representative of other socioeconomic, racial or ethnic, or age groups of lesbians.

4. The lack of appropriate control or comparison groups makes it difficult to assess the health of lesbians relative to other groups of women. In many research designs it may be useful to compare lesbians to another subgroup of women (e.g., heterosexual women, women in general). However, few studies have allowed direct comparisons between lesbians and other subgroups of women by using the same sampling strategies to identify subjects across sexual orientations and including measures of sexual orientation. Some studies have used as a comparison findings from earlier studies of women randomly selected from the general population. Although this method is an improvement on having no comparison group, the two groups are often quite different in terms of several key demographic variables. For example, most studies of lesbian health have included women who are more highly educated, of higher socioeconomic status, younger, and more predominately white compared to probability samples of women in general. In addition, it is important to note that samples from the general population of women include some unknown percentage of lesbians whose results affect the general population findings in undetermined ways.

In selecting a sample comparison group, it could be useful to consider some of the matching strategies commonly used in epidemiological case-control studies where the intent is to sample a control group that is similar to the case group on one or more specified characteristics. In applying these general principles from epidemiology, the comparison group of women could be matched to the lesbians on a pairwise or groupwise basis. Some lesbian health studies are using this approach by defining the comparison group of women as a sister, work colleague, or neighbor of the lesbian research participant.

5. The lack of longitudinal data limits understanding of lesbian development and its implications for how to define and measure lesbian sexual orientation. Most existing studies portray cross sections of experience at one point in time, rather than development over time. Although discontinuity and change characterize the lives of many lesbians, the available cross-sectional data cannot address compelling questions of behavior and identity across time. Prospective, longitudinal studies are essential for understanding vulnerability, resilience, and well-being of lesbians across their life span.

In the following sections, several key methodological issues in conducting research on lesbian health are discussed briefly: defining and sampling the study population, developing instruments to assess being lesbian, and eliciting disclosure of information.[1]

---

[1]The research design and data collection issues involved in conducting research on sexual behavior were addressed more comprehensively by the National Research Council Committee on AIDS Research and the Behavioral, Social, and Statistical Sciences (NRC, 1989, 1990). The reader is also referred to Bradburn et al. (1979) for a more detailed discussion of response effects to threatening questions in survey research and strategies for improving interview methods and questionnaire design.

An in-depth discussion of the methodological issues in conducting research on lesbian health is beyond the scope and resources of this workshop study. The intent of the committee is to highlight the range of issues involved in doing research with lesbians and to suggest some approaches for addressing them. Numerous books on research design and methodology are available that provide more detailed and technical analyses of these issues.

DEFINING THE POPULATION

A critical initial step in conducting research is to clearly specify the target population you wish to study. To sample and identify the lesbian study population, researchers must thus clarify how they have defined sexual orientation in terms of identity, behavior, attraction or desire, or some combination of these. The type of question (e.g., identity versus behavior versus attraction) should be driven by the hypotheses being assessed. Thus, if one wishes to do a study of women who describe themselves as lesbian, perhaps to explore the process of coming out to family members, it may be sufficient to ask a single question such as, Do you consider yourself to be a lesbian? Women who answer yes can then be considered eligible respondents or subjects. In another instance where one wishes to study, for example, woman-to-woman transmission of a sexually transmitted disease, this question would not be a very appropriate strategy for identifying eligible participants. Some women who self-identify as lesbians and would thus qualify for the first study would not fit parameters of the transmission study because they have never had sex with a woman, they may be in an active sexual relationship with a man, or they are not sexually active.

Definitions of the lesbian population and assumptions about its composition and behavior have varied in this body of research, a characteristic also of research on gay men and homosexuality in general. A review by Sell and Petrulio (1996) of 152 public health articles published between 1990 and 1992 that included gay men or lesbians revealed that only four of the studies reported the conceptual definition of sexual orientation employed to identify the population sampled (e.g., indicating that they defined homosexuality in terms of sexual behavior or attraction). The remaining studies typically relied on self-identification to define subjects or defined their sample based on the setting from which it was obtained (e.g., gay and lesbian organizations, bars, clinical settings). Table 3.1 presents information about the way in which lesbian sexual orientation has been defined in a wide range of studies. As illustrated in the table, specific questions have varied across studies, and studies have focused on different components of sexual orientation.

> *We found that there were just so many different varieties of combinations of self-identification, of attraction to women and men, and sexual behavior, either current sexual behavior or past sexual behavior, that well over 30 different groups were defined by the combination of those variables.*

> Alice Dan, Public Workshop, October 6–7, 1997
> Washington, D.C.

INSTRUMENTATION

There are no agreed-upon standard questions with which to assess whether or not a woman is a lesbian (see Chapter 1). Once researchers wishing to assess sexual orientation determine *which* dimensions or aspects of sexual orientation are most relevant to the study, they must then decide *how* to measure the chosen dimensions.

Researchers have used an array of questions to identity lesbians, focusing on the different components of lesbian sexual orientation: self-identification, sexual behavior, or sexual attraction or desire. Further, there is variation in the time periods during which the different components were assessed (e.g., lifetime or recently). However, there are no standard questions for measuring these dimensions. Thus, in one study, women might be identified as lesbian if they had had *only* female sex partners during their lifetime; in another study, women might be identified as lesbian if they had had *any* female sex partners during the past five years. This lack of standardization has made it very difficult to compare results across studies. Sell and Petrulio (1996) found that self-reported lesbian, homosexual, or bisexual identity was by far the most common method used to categorize lesbians in public health research in the studies they surveyed (see Table 3.2).

The committee does not believe that enough information is available at this time to determine what, if any, particular wording is best in questions designed to elicit information about various aspects of sexual orientation. Methodological research is needed to improve measurement

TABLE 3.1 Summary of Measures of Sexual Orientation Used in Studies of Lesbian Health

Study	Measures Used to Assess Sexual Orientation	
	Identity	Behavior
Berger et al., 1995		Sexually active during lifetime with one or more female partners; no sexual intercourse with men during past 12 months
Bevier et al., 1995		Sex of sexual partners since 1978; engagement in vaginal intercourse, oral–penile sex, and/or anal intercourse in more than 50% of sexual encounters
Bloomfield, 1993	Whether women report being primarily heterosexual, primarily or exclusively lesbian, or bisexual	
Brand et al., 1992	Scale from 1 = exclusively heterosexual to 5 = exclusively gay or lesbian	
with weight, and exercise activity (*n* = 124)		
Buenting, 1992		
Carroll et al., 1997	Self-identification as lesbian, bisexual, hetero-sexual, or other	Sex of partner asked with respect to participation in nine specific sexual practices; years since last male sexual encounter; lifetime number of male and female partners
Chicago Women's Health Study (Hughes et al., 1997)	Self-identification: "only heterosexual, mostly heterosexual, bisexual, mostly homosexual, or only homosexual"	Sexual behavior in the past year: "only men, mostly men, equally men and women, mostly women, only women"

Desire	Focus of Study (sample size)
	Whether bacterial vaginosis occurs in lesbians and, if it does, whether it is sexually transmitted ($n = 103$)
	Characteristics, behaviors, and HIV infection of women attending an STD[a] clinic who reported same-sex contact ($n = 135$) compared to women who had sex only with men ($n = 1,383$)
	Drinking patterns of self-identified heterosexual women and self-identified lesbian or bisexual women in San Francisco ($n = 844$)
	Comparison of lesbians, gay men, and heterosexuals on weight, dieting, preoccupation with weight, and exercise activity ($n = 124$)
Sex of preferred sexual partner	Survey of health lifestyles of lesbian and heterosexual women ($n = 79$)
	STD testing, diagnosis, and sexual practices among self-identified lesbian and bisexual women ($n = 421$)
Current sexual interest or attraction: "only men, mostly men, equally men and women, mostly women, only women"	Indicators of mental health in lesbians ($n = 284$) and a comparison group of heterosexual women ($n = 134$)

Continued

TABLE 3.1 *Continued*

| | Measures Used to Assess Sexual Orientation | |
| Study | Identity | Behavior |

Study	Identity	Behavior
Chu et al., 1990		"After 1977 and preceding the diagnosis of AIDS, did this patient have sexual relations with a male partner?" "After 1977 and preceding the diagnosis of AIDS, did this patient have sexual relations with a female partner?" If only female partners, then classified as lesbian; if both male and female partners, then bisexual
Deren et al., 1996	"Do you consider yourself to be hetero-sexual [straight], lesbian, bisexual, other?"	Sex of sexual partner(s) during past 30 days (men only, women only, women and men)
Einhorn and Polgar, 1994	Self-defined as lesbians, bisexual, or undefined	Sex of sexual partners since 1978
Turner et al., 1998b		Whether engaged in woman-to-woman sex during period between consecutive interviews or blood samples (approximately 6 months)
Gómez et al., 1996	"What do you consider your sexual orientation to be?"	"How many women, in total, have you had sex with in the past 3 years?" "In the past 3 years, how many men have you had sex with?"

Desire	Focus of Study (sample size)
	Assess demographic characteristics and behavioral risk factors in lesbians in national surveillance data for reported cases of AIDS ($n = 79$)
	Relationship of sexual orientation to HIV risk behavior and serostatus in a multisite sample of drug-injecting and crack-using women ($n = 830$ lesbians; $n = 5,791$ heterosexual women)
	HIV risk behavior among lesbians and bisexual women ($n = 1,086$)
	Assess HIV status in male and female out-of-treatment drug injectors to determine risk factors for HIV seroconversion in high- and low-seroprevalence cities ($n = 6,882$)
	Risk for HIV and other STDs in order to develop relevant prevention strategies ($n = 461$)

Continued

TABLE 3.1 *Continued*

	Measures Used to Assess Sexual Orientation	
Study	Identity	Behavior
Johnson et al., 1987	Categorize self as lesbian, bisexual, or heterosexual	Lifetime history of hetero-sexual intercourse (0, 1–9, 10–100, or >100 episodes)
Krieger and Sidney, 1997	"Have you experienced discrimination, been prevented from doing something, or been hassled or made to feel inferior in any of the following situations because of your sexual preference (heterosexual, bisexual, homosexual)? (yes or no) a. In your family; b. at school; c. getting a job; d. at work; e. at home"	Lifetime number of same- and other-sex sexual partners
Lemp et al., 1995	Self-reported lesbian or bisexual identity	Sex of sexual partners since 1978 (men only, men and women, women only); engagement in specific sexual behaviors (e.g., oral sex with women)
Michigan Lesbian Health Survey (Bybee and Roeder, 1990)	7-point scale: "Circle the number below that best describes how you think of yourself" Lesbian = 1; 4 = bisexual; heterosexual only = 7	Whether ever had sexual contact with a woman; number of female sexual partners in the past year; whether ever had sex with a man; time since most recent sexual contact with a man; age at first sexual experience with a woman.

Desire	Focus of Study (sample size)
	Reproductive system problems of lesbian and bisexual women in a nonclinical setting ($n = 1,921$ lesbians; $n = 424$ bisexual women)
	Prevalence of self-reported experiences of discrimination based on sexual orientation among black and white adults with same-sex sexual partners, and health-related consequences of discrimination ($n = 1,724$; $n = 1,031$ women; $n = 114$ lesbian or bisexual women)
	HIV seroprevalence and risk behaviors among lesbians and bisexual women in San Francisco and Berkeley ($n = 550$)
	General health and HIV risk of lesbians across the state of Michigan ($n = 1,681$)

Continued

TABLE 3.1 *Continued*

	Measures Used to Assess Sexual Orientation	
Study	Identity	Behavior
National Black Lesbian Study (Cochran and Mays, 1988, 1994; Cochran et al., 1996)	Whether consider self gay or lesbian, bisexual, or neither, but homosexually active	Number of female sexual partners; whether have ever had heterosexual sexual intercourse, time since last previous heterosexual experience; whether currently heterosexually active "never," "rarely," "sometimes," or "regularly"
National Health and Social Life Survey (Laumann et al., 1994)	"Do you think of yourself as heterosexual, homosexual, bisexual, or something else?"	During the past 12 months, past 5 years, and since turning age 18, what was sex of sexual partner(s); how many male and female partners; whether engaged in specific sexual acts: "Now I would like to ask you some questions about sexual experience with females after you were 12 or 13, that is, after puberty. How old were you the first time you had sex with a female?"
National Lesbian Health Care Survey (Bradford and Ryan, 1988)	7-point scale: "Please circle the number on the line below that best describes how you think of yourself." 1 = lesbian only; 4 = bisexual; 7 = heterosexual only	"Describe your past and present situations: in a tight committed primary relationship with a woman; single, but somewhat involved with a woman; single, not involved with anyone; living with a male lover; legally married to a man"; "How old were you when you first had sex with a woman?"

Desire	Focus of Study (sample size)
	Health of African-American women in the United States who have sex with women (*n* = 605)
"On a scale of 1 to 4, where 1 is very appealing and 4 is not at all appealing, how would you rate each of these activities: having sex with someone of the same sex?" "In general, are you sexually attracted to only men, mostly men, both men and women, mostly women, only women?"	Sexual behaviors and practices of Americans (*n* = 3,432 total men and women; *n* = 1,749 women; *n* = 150 women reporting any same-gender sexuality)
	Health and mental health status and needs of U.S. lesbians (*n* = 1,925)

Continued

TABLE 3.1 *Continued*

| Study | Measures Used to Assess Sexual Orientation | |
	Identity	Behavior
Norman et al., 1996	5-point scale: exclusively heterosexual, primarily heterosexual, bisexual, primarily homosexual, exclusively homosexual	Number of male and female partners during past 2 months with whom engaged in particular sexual practices; number of times engaged in such practices
Nurses' Study II Pilot Study (Case, 1996; Case et al., 1996)	"Whether you are sexually active or not, what is your sexual identity or orientation? Heterosexual; bisexual; lesbian, gay, or homosexual; none of the above; prefer not to answer"	
Robertson and Schachter, 1981		Whether sexually active with only women during the past 6 months
Russell et al., 1995	Indicate whether heterosexual, homosexual, lesbian, or bisexual	"Have you had any of the following forms of sexual contact in the past 2 weeks? 1. Between your mouth and a partner's penis? 2. Between your mouth and a partner's vulva/vagina? 3. Between your mouth and a partner's anus?"
Shaffer et al., 1995	"Did she describe herself as gay/bisexual?"	"Did she ever have a homosexual experience?"

Desire	Focus of Study (sample size)
	Risk for HIV infection of lesbian and bisexual women residing in small cities ($n = 1,057$)
	Longitudinal study of health status and behaviors of a national cohort of registered nurses ($n = 1,050$ in pilot study)
	Screening of sexually active lesbians for STDs ($n = 148$)
	Presence of sexually transmitted pharyngeal bacteria and carriage rate in sexually active adults attending a genitourinary clinic ($n = 492$ heterosexual women; $n = 41$ lesbians; $n = 9$ bisexual women; $n = 586$ men)
	Use of psychological autopsies of adolescents who had committed suicide to examine relationship between sexual orientation and suicide ($n = 120$)

Continued

TABLE 3.1 *Continued*

	Measures Used to Assess Sexual Orientation	
Study	Identity	Behavior
Smith et al., 1985	"When did you first consider yourself to be a lesbian?" "Do you consider yourself to be bisexual?"	7-point Kinsey scale[b]
Trevathan et al., 1993		Evidence of intimate contact between the members of the dyad (sleeping in the same bed or sexual interaction reported on the daily checklists); no sleeping or sex with men reported on the daily checklists
Women's Health Initiative (The Women's Health Initiative Study Group, 1998)		"Regardless of whether you are currently sexually active, which response *best describes* who you have had sex with over your adult lifetime: 1) have never had sex; 2) sex with a woman or with women; 3) sex with a man or with men; 4) sex with both men and women; 5) prefer not to answer" If option 4 selected, then "Which response *best describes* who you have had sex with after 45 years of age? 0) never had sex 1) sex with a woman or with women; 2) sex with a man or with men; 3) sex with both men and women"

NOTE: Reports of studies rarely include the exact wording of the questions used to determine sexual orientation. Where this information is available, it is included in the table. Otherwise, the questions are described as in the report of research results.

Desire	Focus of Study (sample size)
7-point Kinsey scale[b]	Experiences during gynecologic care, sources of care, and utilization patterns of lesbian and bisexual women (n = 424 bisexual women; n = 1,921 lesbians)
	Menstrual synchrony in lesbian couples (n = 29 couples)
	Strategies for the prevention and control of common causes of morbidity and mortality among postmenopausal women, including cancer, cardiovascular disease, and osteoporosis-related fractures (n = 64,500 women in the clinical trial; n = 100,000 women in the observational study only)

[a]STD = sexually transmitted disease.

[b]The Kinsey scale (NRC, 1997) of sexual orientation rates sexual orientation on a 7-point scale with 0 = exclusively heterosexual behavior and attraction and 6 = exclusively homosexual behavior and attraction. The scale does not separate behavior and attraction.

TABLE 3.2 Operational Methods of Identifying Subjects in Public Health Research, 1990–1992

Operational Method	Percent*
Self-reported identity	64.6
Setting (e.g., lesbian bar)	29.2
Sexual history	4.2
Kinsey scale	6.2
Other scale	16.7

*Categories total more than 100% because some studies used more than one method. Data are included from 48 studies that categorized women as homosexual, lesbian, or bisexual.
SOURCE: Adapted from Sell and Petrulio, 1996.

of various dimensions of lesbian sexual orientation. It is particularly important to discover how best to measure these dimensions among women of different racial and ethnic backgrounds, birth cohorts, religious backgrounds, and social classes. This should include qualitative studies—among them, ethnographic research—to better understand how a lesbian sexual orientation is defined in different subgroups of lesbians. In light of the current lack of information for better defining a lesbian sexual orientation, the committee believes that researchers of lesbian health should take care to clearly state the reasons they selected particular questions for their study and, where possible, should use questions whose wording has already been tested in comparable studies, particularly such large-scale studies as the Nurses' Health Study II (NHS-II) and the Women's Health Initiative (WHI).

DISCLOSURE OF SEXUAL ORIENTATION[2]

In order to identify lesbians in a sample, respondents to study questions must be willing to disclose information about their sexual orientation and sexual behaviors. An important challenge for researchers on les-

---

[2]This section incorporates portions of the workshop presentation of Dr. Charles Turner.

bian health is to design instruments and strategies that increase the chances that women will reveal this kind of sensitive information about themselves. It is, of course, important to ensure confidentiality in surveys of lesbian health whether or not the surveys are anonymous (see Chapter 4). However, even when precautions have been taken to ensure that confidentiality will be maintained, respondents may remain distrustful. If respondents do not believe and trust the researcher, they are unlikely to respond honestly to sensitive questions.

Methods to Increase Disclosure

People's willingness to disclose sensitive information about themselves can be influenced by the methods used to elicit the information. For example, in a large-scale field experiment that included measures of self-reported drug use, respondents revealed more information about their drug use on a self-administered paper-and-pencil form than when they were questioned by an interviewer (Turner et al., 1992). These differences in reporting became more pronounced as the sensitivity of the information increased (e.g., cocaine use compared to alcohol use, a more socially accepted behavior). However, although this information might suggest that self-administered questionnaires should always be used, since all respondents do not have the appropriate level of literacy to understand and answer the questions, this method can also lead to substantial amounts of total or item nonresponse.[3]

New techniques have been developed to increase the likelihood that respondents will report sensitive behaviors. One promising technology is the audio computer-assisted self-interview (audio-CASI) in which questions are asked of the respondent by using digitized audio files of a human voice, rather than a human interviewer, and the subject responds using a computer keyboard. A major advantage of using audio-CASI is that it provides fully private administration in a completely standardized interview situation. Additionally, respondents do not have to be literate. Al-

---

[3]Total nonresponse occurs when the subject answers *no* items on a questionnaire; item nonresponse occurs when a respondent who answers most of the questions does not respond to a particular item.

though they must be able to use a computer keyboard, this has not been a big problem, even in studies of special populations such as elderly mono-lingual Koreans surveyed by monolingual English-speaking interviewers (Hendershot et al., 1996).

The audio-CASI method can also be employed over the telephone (telephone audio-CASI, or T-ACASI). This approach, in which respondents actually respond to a computer, can be set up as a call-in program, so that in a prospective study, respondents can be scheduled to call every week to report on the behaviors of interest (e.g., sensitive health behaviors). Follow-ups can then be done with those who fail to keep these appointments. To maximize the representativeness of the sample the research project should be prepared to supply the required touch-tone phones to the few participants who do not have them.

Studies using the audio-CASI method have found that people are much more likely to reveal sensitive information about themselves (e.g., sexual difficulties) than they would if responding to a human interviewer. For example, in the National Survey of Adolescent Males, which is a national probability sample of 15- to 19-year-old males, respondents were almost four times as likely to report some type of male-to-male sexual contact when the audio-CASI method was used rather than a self-administered paper questionnaire (Turner et al., 1998b). This pattern of higher rates of reported behaviors when using the CASI mode was true for specific sexual acts as well.[4]

In a pilot study described at the workshop (Turner, 1997), male participants were randomly assigned to one of two conditions for gathering their responses to questions on high-risk sexual behavior: punching buttons on their touch-tone phones or reporting in to an interviewer. Those using the telephone punch button method were much more likely to reveal higher levels of more sensitive behaviors (e.g., more anal sex, less condom use) and to report having had sex fewer than ten times in the last six months.

---

[4] Respondents were asked whether they had ever engaged in such male-to-male sexual contacts as mutual masturbation; receptive or insertive oral sex; or, receptive or insertive anal sex. For the individual behaviors assessed, crude odds ratios ranged from 1.9 to 7.9, and adjusted odds ratios from 2.3 to 7.9, for the alternate estimates of prevalence using different methods of questioning, with higher estimates obtained using CASI methods (Turner et al., 1998b). Odds were adjusted for race, age, whether ever had sexual intercourse with a female, and health insurance status.

These technologies have been field-tested in other groups. In the 1995 Survey of Family Growth (Mosher and Duffer, 1995), 10,000 females were asked questions about their history of abortions and other sensitive topics using both audio-CASI and interviewer questioning. Women in this survey reported significantly more abortions when questioned by using audio-CASI (Miller et al., in press). Similarly, in the Gay Urban Men Survey (Turner et al., 1998a) a randomly selected subset of respondents answered questions using T-ACASI.

There has been some suggestion that computer-assisted techniques will not be well accepted among lesbians. Interestingly, although the same concerns were voiced about using this technology with gay men, it has now been employed quite successfully in studies of this population (Turner, 1997). Additional testing will be needed to determine whether this is, in fact, a useful technology in studies of lesbians.

SAMPLING[5]

Sampling is the method by which subjects are selected from a target population. Subpopulation subgroups that represent only a small proportion of the general population present significant challenges for probability sampling (Kalton, 1993). The challenge of sampling rare population subgroups such as lesbians is to find economical methods for obtaining the sample (Kalton, 1993). This is even more difficult in the case of lesbians because they are a stigmatized group and are not readily identifiable.

When developing sampling strategies it is important to keep in mind that lesbians are not a homogeneous population. The samples in most lesbian health research to date can be characterized as primarily white, relatively well-educated, middle-class, young adults who identify themselves as lesbians (Greene, 1994; Rankow, 1995; Trippet, 1994). Few studies have captured the diversity of the experiences of lesbians across race, culture, socioeconomic spheres, age, and time. In particular, few studies have attempted to explicitly sample racial or ethnic minority groups

---

[5]This section incorporates significant portions of the testimony presented by Drs. Susan Cochran and Graham Kalton.

such as African Americans, Latinos, or Asians, or to sample across the socioeconomic spectrum. To obtain representative samples, however, research sampling plans must take care to include all appropriate segments of these communities.

In the following sections, several different approaches to sampling rare populations are considered for their applicability to research with lesbians. The section begins with a discussion of probability sampling and nonprobability sampling, and follows with descriptions of probability sampling techniques that can be used to identify a sample. Certain of these sampling strategies hold potential for improving research on lesbian issues; others are not yet practical. Some studies use only one of these methods to select a sample; others incorporate several methods into the research sampling plan.

Probability Sampling

In a probability-based design, individuals in the population (in this case, the population of lesbians) are enumerated in some fashion and a sample is then selected. Ideally, to conduct population-based sampling the population of interest (the target population) is clearly defined and identifiable. Researchers have a means of reaching out to each and every member of the population, and the probability of selecting each potential respondent is known. If all of these sampling conditions are met and there is a high response rate, then the prevalence of a risk factor or an outcome in a sample can be generalized confidently to the population as a whole. In practice, however, such ideal conditions are rarely met. Probability sampling has rarely been used in studies of lesbian health.

The population-based sampling frame most likely to be useful for lesbians would be to sample women in general and collect information to identify a lesbian subsample. However, most probability sampling designs are extremely difficult to use with the lesbian population for three important reasons:

1. Lesbians represent a hidden population. Lesbians do not represent a readily visible population. Many lesbians are reluctant to disclose their sexual orientation for fear of stigmatization, discrimination, or other negative impact. Thus, it can be very difficult to identify lesbians in the population.

2. Lesbians tend to be a geographically dispersed population. Lesbians live in all parts of the country, in both urban and rural areas, and in all types of communities. Although communities can be identified in most large cities where high concentrations of gay men reside, lesbians have been less likely to live in these or similar areas. Thus, it can be extremely difficult to locate the population from which to draw a sample.

3. Lesbians represent only a small minority of women. Because lesbians represent only a small percentage of the population, the overall sample of women must be very large to identify a large enough subsample of lesbians for meaningful analyses. For example, if lesbians represent 2 to 3% of women, then drawing an overall sample of 1,000 women would be expected to yield a subsample of only 20 to 30 lesbians, too few for most analytic purposes. As noted before, adding sexual orientation questions to large population-based surveys (e.g., the National Health and Nutrition Examination Survey [NHANES] or the National Health Interview Survey [NHIS]), is one possible option for identifying larger probability-based samples of lesbians.

Nonprobability Sampling

Sample surveys on lesbian health have most commonly used nonprobability sampling. Unlike probability sampling, in nonprobability designs the probability of selecting any one individual is unknown. Because the effects of potential bias cannot be determined with nonprobability samples, observed prevalences and relationships may or may not reflect those existing in the lesbian population as a whole.

Nonprobability samples are always vulnerable to selection bias, but the nature of this bias can change over time. For example, several decades ago, because social scientists and psychiatrists presumed that homosexuality represented psychopathology, it was believed reasonable to look for lesbians in psychiatric settings. Not surprisingly, these researchers found a high prevalence of psychiatric problems in their lesbian subjects. In a wave of social science research beginning in the 1970s, researchers looked for their samples in sites where lesbians obviously congregated, such as bars or feminist and lesbian activist meetings. Not surprisingly, scientists found in those samples that lesbians consumed alcohol and, parenthetically, were predominantly feminists and lesbian activists. This confounding of outcome variables with convenience sampling strategies undermines confidence in the prevalences of particular behaviors, health risks, and health and mental health conditions reported in these studies.

Much of the existing research on lesbians has obtained research subjects from lesbian community groups (e.g., mailing or membership lists from lesbian or gay organizations). Other researchers have obtained subjects at regional or national gay or lesbian events that draw people from a large geographic area. These nonprobability methods of obtaining lesbian research subjects yield samples that are not representative of the general population of lesbians since they are limited to lesbians who are open enough about their sexual orientation to attend community events or who subscribe to lesbian and gay newspapers and magazines.

These sampling biases may not be fatal flaws, however, if the researcher's interest is in a particular subset of the lesbian population. For example, a sample drawn at a widely attended lesbian event may be relatively representative of lesbians who have come out, a potentially important group for researchers to study because they are the most visible to the public and so may affect how heterosexuals view lesbians. Therefore, nonprobability samples can generate population estimates that may be generalizable to restricted subpopulations of lesbians. It is critical, however, that the limits of generalization be acknowledged and that the findings observed in these restricted groups are *not* assumed to apply to all lesbians. For many purposes of health research, however, such as measuring the prevalence of disease conditions or risk factors in lesbians, more representative sampling designs will be preferable to nonprobability samples.

Sampling Techniques

A variety of sampling techniques have been designed to identify members of "rare" population subgroups for research studies (i.e., subgroups which comprise a small percentage of the general population).[6] Probability sampling techniques include one-stage screening and two-phase screening, disproportionate stratification, multiple frames, and multiplicity sampling. Nonprobability sampling techniques include location (or convenience) sampling and snowball sampling. The possible uses of these methods to select samples of lesbians are described in the following sections.

One-Stage Screening and Two-Phase Screening

The most straightforward method of sampling a rare population subgroup is to take a sample of the total population and screen out everybody who is *not* a member of this population subgroup. The amount of screening necessary depends on the prevalence of the population subgroup of interest. For example, to obtain a sample of 1,000 members of a population subgroup with a prevalence rate of 10%, 10,000 people will have to be screened. If the prevalence is 5%, 20,000 people will have to be screened, and so forth. Clearly, this strategy can become very expensive if face-to-face interviews are used; less expensive alternatives include telephone interviews and mail questionnaires.

A possible application of one-stage screening would be to sample from communities in which lesbians are known to live, such as North Hampton, Massachusetts, or some neighborhoods in San Francisco. In these areas, the density of lesbian residents might be high enough to make initial household screening economically feasible, particularly by telephone. Unfortunately, the focus on these geographical areas, although it solves the problem of economically feasible enumeration, also introduces significant selection bias because lesbians who reside in high-density lesbian

---

[6]Researchers have developed a number of innovative strategies to sample rare and/or difficult-to-identify populations. For example, people who are homeless represent an example of another difficult-to-identify subpopulation for which there is a lack of agreed-upon definition. Rossi et al. (1987) attempted to enumerate literally homeless individuals in Chicago by both taking a probability sample of individuals spending the night in homeless shelters and conducting a complete enumeration of people encountered in a thorough search of non-dwelling unit places in a probability sample of census blocks.

neighborhoods are not likely to be representative of the lesbian population as a whole.

A two-phase screening procedure can be used when it is expensive or difficult to screen for a member of a rare population subgroup. In this case, a few questions are asked in the first phase of screening to quickly identify either households likely to contain lesbians or individuals likely to be lesbian. Then, only these households or persons are asked more detailed screening questions in the second stage to determine which individuals actually are lesbian. However, this two-phase strategy is useful only if two conditions apply: (1) the first phase of screening must be much cheaper than the second; (2) the first-phase screening process must not screen out many women who actually *are* lesbian.

These strategies obviously depend on the willingness of lesbians to disclose their sexual orientation in the screening interview. Depending on the sampling strategies used, there is also a risk that some desired subgroups of the lesbian population will be excluded. In the case of telephone survey sampling of lesbians (e.g., using random digit dialing), there is a risk that individuals will be missed who live in nontelephone households, which is disproportionally true of poor households, as well as those in institutions, those who are homeless, and so on. Methodological research needs to be conducted to determine the feasibility of using screening methods to identify samples of lesbians and to assess the effects of possible bias.

Disproportionate Stratification

In disproportionate stratification, some part of the general population in which the population of interest is concentrated is identified and oversampled (i.e., sampled with a higher probability than the rest of the population). The geographic areas in which a population subgroup tends to be concentrated are placed in one stratum and all other geographic areas in another stratum. In other words, areas where high concentrations of lesbians reside are identified and the "lesbian-rich" stratum is then oversampled.

There are a variety of methods for identifying a sampling stratum in which population subgroups are concentrated. For example, the Gay Urban Men Study (also known as the Multicultural Men's Health Survey), which is selecting a probability sample of gay and bisexual men in 10 large cities, employed such sources as census information on households with two adult male unmarried partners, local informants, membership lists, and commercial marketing lists to identify geographic areas with high concentrations of gay men (Binson et al., 1996). The researchers note that these methods have some inherent biases: they are more likely to identify those who self-identify as gay or bisexual, and they will be less likely to sample those who have same-sex partners but do not identify as gay or bisexual.

For a disproportionate stratification strategy to work effectively, two conditions—which rarely occur together—must be met. First, there must be a much higher prevalence of the population subgroup of interest (e.g., lesbians) in the geographic area where it is believed to be concentrated. Secondly, this geographic area also has to contain a high proportion of the population subgroup. Although there are potential gains from using this form of oversampling, they are limited because lesbians may not be concentrated in particular geographic areas, and even if they are, the areas may not contain a large percentage of the total lesbian population. Further, lesbians who do choose to live in areas where lesbians are concentrated are likely not representative of the lesbian population in general, although the analyses can in part be corrected for this by weighting the sample to get the proper representation. Also, in some cases, this strategy can be more costly than alternatively taking a large enough random sample to reach the desired sample size.

Multiple Frames

If no one sampling frame gives adequate coverage of the population subgroup of interest, a combination of frames may be used. For example, household sampling may be combined with membership lists of one or more lesbian organizations to increase the number of lesbians in the sample. A risk with this approach, however, is that individuals will appear on more than one of the sampling lists or frames, thus increasing their chances of being selected into the sample. This issue can be addressed by collating the multiple lists or frames and then eliminating duplicates before drawing the sample or by weighting responses in the analyses to adjust for the chances that names on one list are duplicated on another.

Multiplicity or Network Sampling

The goal of multiplicity or network sampling is to reduce the amount of screening necessary to identify members of the population subgroup by capitalizing on linkages to relatives or neighbors. Its most likely use is to estimate the size of a hard-to-identify population subgroup.[7] With this strategy, an interviewed subject is asked to identify others (e.g., relatives or neighbors) who are members of the population subgroup and, in some cases, to provide data on them. This method requires that respondents be able and willing to report whether people linked to them are members of the population subgroup. Further, if the characteristics of the population subgroup are being studied, the respondents must be able to report on these characteristics accurately, or the individuals they identify must be contacted in person and interviewed. If multiple routes of sample selection are used, responses must be weighted in the analyses to compensate for differential probabilities of selection. There are clearly both ethical and logistical problems in using this technique to estimate the number of lesbians or to obtain samples of lesbians. First, lesbians' sexual orientation may not be known to all others in their networks and so they would not be identified. Second, even if a lesbian's sexual orientation is known to the respondent, she may not want the respondent to disclose this information to others.

---

[7]Killworth et al. (1998) describe the use of a social network approach to estimate the size of hard-to-count populations. In their study, a representative sample of the U.S. population was asked how many people they knew in 29 populations of known size, and how many people they knew in 3 populations of unknown size whose size the researchers wanted to estimate (people who are homeless, women who were raped in the past 12 months, and people who are HIV-positive). Responses were then used to calculate a maximum likelihood estimate of the number of people in the respondent's social network, and the patterns of all respondents' responses about the populations of unknown size were used to estimate the size of the unknown subpopulations. The method accurately estimated the size of 20 of the 29 known populations, and the calculated estimates of the unknown populations were consistent with other published estimates. To the committee's knowledge, this approach has not yet been used to estimate the size of the lesbian population, but it is a strategy that might yield useful information.

Snowball Sampling

In snowball sampling, members of a population subgroup are identified and asked to identify or report on other members of the population subgroup. The chances of being identified thus depend to some extent on the level of involvement in various social and community networks. Once a list or frame is obtained that contains all or a large proportion of the population subgroup, it is possible to draw a probability sample from the list. It is important that the snowball technique not simply be stopped when a desired sample size is reached. Rather, snowball sampling should be continued until a full roster of names believed to contain a large percentage of the population of interest is developed; then individuals from this list can be randomly sampled into the study.

Although snowballing can be useful for constructing a sampling frame of all members of some population subgroups, given the hidden nature of the lesbian population and the potential risks of disclosure, it is not likely to be a feasible strategy for use with this population.

Location (Convenience) Sampling

In location sampling, sometimes referred to as convenience sampling, members of a rare population are sampled in places where they congregate, for example, gay bars or bookstores, where there is a high expectation of sufficient lesbian density to make the sampling efficient. Unfortunately, this strategy, too, results in significant sampling bias because bars are more likely to be frequented by young women who are old enough to drink and by women who drink more frequently, just as lesbian bookstores might be visited more frequently by feminists, and so forth.

One suggested strategy for improving location sampling is first to map all of the possible sites and then to draw samples from within these sites in ways that cover multiple time periods and geographic areas. There are, nevertheless, significant problems with this methodology. First, only people who go to these particular sites (e.g., bars or bookstores) will be sampled. Second, people who go to these sites more frequently have a greater probability of being selected into the sample. Thus, the location sampling method produces a probability sample of visits rather than visitors.

Combining Strategies for Sampling Lesbians

Many lesbian health research studies have used nonprobability sampling that goes far beyond convenience sampling, employing multiple methods in an attempt to obtain more broadly representative samples in a geographic area (e.g., sampling from newsletter rosters, women in gay and lesbian bookstores, lesbian community organizations, attendees at women's music festivals). Each of these methods casts the net wider and wider, attempting to sample participants from outside the social networks of the researcher or from outside institutional settings such as clinics and hospitals. Nonetheless, no matter how wide the net becomes, these methods are all still non-probability-based sample designs and are subject to criticism for selection bias even if they represent the most sophisticated methods now used in lesbian research.

Given the difficulties in conducting population-based probability sampling of lesbians and the cost-efficiency of non-probability-based designs, an important research question is whether techniques can be employed to improve the usefulness of non-probability-based samples. One strategy might be to examine the consistency of findings across studies that use different sampling methods across different settings, with the expectation that results might center around the true population parameter. Confidence in reported estimates can increase as replicated well-designed studies are published on lesbian health using similar variables.

ADDING SEXUAL ORIENTATION QUESTIONS TO EXISTING STUDIES

One suggestion for increasing the amount of information on lesbian health is to add sexual orientation items to large sample surveys or other large studies. This would add a significant amount of analytical capability at little additional cost. Adding appropriate questions about sexual orientation to large cross-sectional or cohort studies strengthens the ability to understand variation in health status by sexual orientation. However, investigators have been reluctant to add such questions to their studies for fear that women would not answer them and, in addition, might be so alienated by the questions that they would not participate in the study. There is evidence, however, that sexual orientation items can be used successfully in studies and in surveys (NRC, 1989).

Two examples of ongoing studies that have included sexual orientation items in their data collection efforts are the Nurses' Health Study II[8,9] and the Women's Health Initiative. In September 1994, NHS-II investigators began to receive requests for information on sexual orientation and health from other researchers and, more importantly, from both lesbian and heterosexual participants in the study itself. In response to these requests, investigators decided to add a question to gather information about sexual identity, hypothesizing that the social experience of women with a lesbian or bisexual sexual orientation might put them at higher risk for a number of conditions, particularly chronic disease and cancer.

Questions were first pilot-tested on a sample of 1,050 nurses for inclusion in the June 1995 questionnaire. A variety of questions were asked in order to compare the willingness of respondents to answer different types, including questions about sexual identity[10] and about the sex of sexual partners over the past five years and during one's lifetime. The researchers found that women were willing to return the form (response rate = 78.4%) and answer the questions on sexual orientation, that they considered these questions acceptable, and that there was little negative feedback.[11] As a result, investigators added a question on sexual identity to the 1995 Nurses' Health Study cohort questionnaire, which was mailed to 116,000 women.

These results must be interpreted with some caution because nurses

---

[8]NHS-II is a prospective cohort of 116,680 female registered nurses established in 1989 as a companion study to the long-running Nurses' Health Study I. Participants are mailed questionnaires every two years that include comprehensive health questions.

[9]The description of the NHS-II is based on the workshop presentation of Dr. Patricia Case.

[10]The item categories included heterosexual; bisexual; lesbian, gay, or homosexual; none of the above; or prefer not to answer.

[11]In the NHS-II pilot study, 98.0% of the respondents reported that they were heterosexual; 0.9% that they were lesbian, gay, or homosexual; and 0.1% that they were bisexual (Case et al., 1996).

may be more willing to respond to questions about sexuality than general population samples. Nonetheless, these results are promising and demonstrate that careful pilot testing of questions in advance can help to reveal patterns of response and ease investigators' fears, often legitimate, of negative effects on the study.

The WHI,[12] a longitudinal study of about 100,000 postmenopausal women, has included one question on its baseline data collection forms about gender of adult lifetime sexual partners (i.e., men, women, both men and women, or never had sex). Questions on sexual orientation could also potentially be added to large national sample surveys such as the Bureau of Labor Statistics National Longitudinal Surveys, NHIS, the NHANES, and the National Survey of Family Growth. Only very large population-based surveys such as these can be expected to yield sufficient sample sizes of lesbians without substantial changes in the existing research design. Consequently, these surveys represent an important opportunity to attempt population-based sampling of lesbians if they were to include questions of sexual orientation. The committee does not believe, however, that it is feasible at this time to add questions regarding sexual orientation to the U.S. Census of Population and Housing for a variety of reasons, including the facts that questions are often asked of one individual in a household who serves as a proxy for the others; that efforts are made to minimize the number of questions, making it difficult to have any kind of item added to the questionnaire; and that the census questions require the approval of the U.S. Congress.

It should be noted that there are also potential drawbacks to the strategy of adding questions to existing surveys. For example, including questions on sexual orientation does not guarantee that they will be considered in the analyses. Alternatively, the data may be analyzed and interpreted by persons who are unfamiliar with the nuances of conducting research with and defining the lesbian population. Another potentially very significant problem is the issue of confidentiality (see Chapter 4). Because these large-scale surveys are confidential but not anonymous, the extent to which lesbians will disclose their sexual orientation in this setting is unclear. Indeed, the degree to which sexual orientation will be

---

[12]See information on WHI in footnote 8 in Chapter 2.

disclosed even when anonymity is ensured is unclear for all studies that inquire about sexual orientation.

AREAS FOR FURTHER METHODOLOGICAL RESEARCH IN STUDYING LESBIAN HEALTH

The committee identified several strategies for increasing the statistical power of research on lesbians. These include pooling data across studies using similar measures and methods; meta-analysis of methodologically sound studies, including those with smaller sample sizes; multisite studies; and fostering national and international collaborations. Nonetheless, the field would benefit greatly from additional research focused on improving research methodologies. This type of research also has significant potential to benefit the conduct of health-related research with other populations, especially other hard-to-identify and/or rare population subgroups.

The committee suggests the following areas for additional research:

1. Research is needed on how techniques for sampling other hard-to-identify and/or rare population subgroups might be applied to obtaining probability samples of lesbians.

2. Research is recommended on the validity and reliability of questions measuring the different dimensions of sexual orientation: identity, behavior, and attraction or desire.

3. Research is needed on technologies to elicit disclosure in order to determine their usefulness in studies with lesbians. It is particularly important to consider how factors such as race and ethnicity, socioeconomic status, age, and region of residence affect the use of such technologies.

4. Qualitative research is needed to increase the depth of understanding of lesbians' lives and to better inform other research. Consideration should be given in larger studies to including experts in qualitative methods in the design team for an integrated approach to seeking information.

5. Existing databases from federal and other large surveys should be reviewed to identify those with potential for analysis by sexual orientation.

6. In the absence of the ability to conduct targeted population-based

studies of lesbians, efforts to create more effective non-probability-based designs should be undertaken.

7. Methodological research is needed on the feasibility of using matched control designs for research directed toward assessing the health status of lesbians compared to other women.

8. There may be innovative ways of sampling that have not been widely used. One suggestion made at the workshop (Gruskin, 1997) is to work with managed care organizations, many of which have research divisions, to obtain samples of lesbians and nonlesbian matched controls. The membership of a managed care organization usually is quite large and captured in a medical care delivery system, and access to information-rich medical records may be possible. Methodological research should be done to investigate the utility of this approach and to examine the ethical issues that it raises, with careful attention to how to maintain confidentiality.

REFERENCES

Berger BJ, Kolton S, Zenilman JM, Cummings MC, Feldman J, McCormack WM. 1995. Bacterial vaginosis in lesbians: A sexually transmitted disease. *Clinical Infectious Diseases* 21(6):1402–1405.

Bevier PJ, Chaisson MA, Hefferman RT, Castro KG. 1995. Women at a sexually transmitted disease clinic who reported same-sex contact: Their HIV seroprevalence and risk behaviors. *American Journal of Public Health* 85(10):1366–1371.

Binson D, Moskowitz TM, Anderson K, Paul J, Stall R, Catania J. 1996. Sampling men who have sex with men: Strategies for a telephone survey in urban areas in the United States. *Proceedings of the Section on Survey Research Methods, American Statistical Association.* Alexandria, VA: American Statistical Association, pp. 68–72.

Bloomfield K. 1993. A comparison of alcohol consumption between lesbians and heterosexual women in an urban population. *Drug and Alcohol Dependence* 33:257–269.

Bradburn NM, Sudman S, Blair E, Locander W, Miles C, Singer E, Stocking C. 1979. *Improving Interview Method and Questionnaire Design.* San Francisco: Jossey-Bass.

Bradford J, Ryan C. 1988. *The National Lesbian Health Care Survey: Final Report.* Washington, DC: National Lesbian and Gay Health Foundation.

Brand PA, Rothblum ED, Solomon LJ. 1992. A comparison of lesbians, gay men, and heterosexuals on weight and restrained eating. *International Journal of Eating Disorders* 11(3):253–259.

Buenting JA. 1992. Health life-styles of lesbian and heterosexual women. Special Issue: Lesbian health: What are the issues? *Health Care for Women International* 13(2):165–171.

Bybee D, Roeder V. 1990. *Michigan Lesbian Health Survey: Results Relevant to AIDS. A Report to the Michigan Organization for Human Rights and the Michigan Department of Public Health.* Lansing: Michigan Department of Health and Human Services.

Carroll N, Goldstein RS, Lo W, Mayer KH. 1997. Gynecological infections and sexual practices of Massachusetts lesbian and bisexual women. *Journal of the Gay and Lesbian Medical Association* 1(1):15–23.

Case P, Spiegelman D, Hunter DJ, Manson JE, Willet WC. 1996. *Sexual Orientation in Relation to Behaviors in the Nurses' Health Study II: Selected Results from a Pilot Study. Presentation to the American Public Health Association.* New York: National Development and Research Institutes.

Chu SY, Buehler JW, Fleming PL, Berkelman RL. 1990. Epidemiology of reported cases of AIDS in lesbians, United States 1980–89. *American Journal of Public Health* 80(11):1380–1381.

Cochran SD, Mays VM. 1988. Disclosure of sexual preference to physicians by black lesbian and bisexual women. *Western Journal of Medicine* 149(5):616–619.

Cochran SD, Bybee D, Gage S, Mays VM. 1996. Prevalence of HIV-related self-reported sexual behaviors, sexually transmitted diseases, and problems with drugs and alcohol in 3 large surveys of lesbian and bisexual women: A look into a segment of the community. *Women's Health Research on Gender, Behavior, and Policy* 2(1–2):11–33.

Deren S, Goldstein M, Williams M, Stark M, Estrada A, Friedman SR, Young RM. 1996. Sexual orientation, HIV risk behavior, and serostatus in a multisite sample of drug-injecting and crack-using women. *Women's Health: Research on Gender, Behavior, and Policy* 2(1–2):35–47.

Einhorn L, Polgar M. 1994. HIV-risk behavior among lesbians and bisexual women. *AIDS Education and Prevention* 6(6):514–523.

Gómez CA, Garcia DR, Kegebein VJ, Shade SB, Hernandez SR. 1996. Sexual identity versus sexual behavior: Implications for HIV prevention strategies for women who have sex with women. *Women's Health: Research on Gender, Behavior, and Policy* 2(1–2):91–109.

Greene B. 1994. Ethnic-minority lesbians and gay men: Mental health and treatment issues. *Journal of Consulting and Clinical Psychology* 62(2):243–251.

Gruskin E. 1997. Presentation before the Institute of Medicine Committee on Lesbian Health Research Priorities. Washington, DC, October 6–7, 1997.

Hendershot TP, Rogers SM, Thornberry JP, Miller HG, Turner CF. 1996. Multilingual audio-CASI: Using English-speaking field interviewers to survey elderly Korean households. In: Warnecke R, ed. *Health Survey Research Methods.* Hyattsville, MD: National Center for Health Statistics.

Hughes TL, Haas AP, Avery L. 1997. Mental health concerns of lesbians: Preliminary results from the Chicago Women's Health Survey. *Journal of the Gay and Lesbian Medical Association* 1(3):137–148.

Hughes TL, Wilsnack SC. 1997. Use of alcohol among lesbians: Research and clinical implications. *American Journal of Orthopsychiatry* 67(1):20–36.

Johnson SR, Smith EM, Guenther SM. 1987. Comparison of gynecologic health care problems between lesbians and bisexual women. A survey of 2,345 women. *Journal of Reproductive Medicine* 32(11):805–811.

Kalton G. 1993. Sampling considerations in research on HIV risk and illness. In: Ostrow DG, Kessler RC, eds. *Methodological Issues in AIDS Behavioral Research.* New York: Plenum Press. Pp. 53–74.

Killworth PD, McCarty C, Bernard HR, Shelley GA, Johnsen EC. 1998. Estimation of seroprevalence, rape, and homelessness in the United States using a social network approach. *Evaluation Review* 22(2):189–308.

Krieger N, Sidney S. 1997. Prevalence and health implications of anti-gay discrimination: A study of black and white women and men in the CARDIA Cohort. *International Journal of Health Services* 27(1):157–176.

Laumann EO, Gagnon JH, Michael RT, Michaels S. 1994. *The Social Organization of Sexuality: Sexual Practices in the United States.* Chicago: University of Chicago Press.

Lemp GF, Jones M, Kellogg TA, Nieri GN, et al. 1995. HIV seroprevalence and risk behaviors among lesbians and bisexual women in San Francisco and Berkeley, California. *American Journal of Public Health* 85(11):1549–1552.

Miller HG, Gribble JN, Rogers SM, Turner CF. In press. Abortion and breast cancer risk: Fact or artifact? In: Stone A, ed. *Science of Self Report (provisional title).* Mahwah, NJ: Lawrence Erlbaum Associates.

Mosher W, Duffer A. 1995. *Innovations in the 1995 National Survey of Family Growth. Paper presented at the annual meeting of the Population Survey of America,* San Francisco, CA.

Norman AD, Perry MJ, Stevenson LY, Kelly JA, Roffman RA. 1996. Lesbian and bisexual women in small cities—At risk for HIV? HIV Prevention Community Collaborative. *Public Health Reports* 111(4):347–352.

NRC (National Research Council). 1989. *AIDS: Sexual Behavior and Intravenous Drug Use.* Washington, DC: National Academy Press.

NRC. 1990. *AIDS: The Second Decade.* Washington, DC: National Academy Press.

NRC. 1997. *Evaluating Genetic Diversity.* Washington, DC: National Academy Press.

Rankow EJ. 1995. Lesbian health issues for the primary care provider. *Journal of Family Practice* 40(5):486–496.

Robertson P, Schachter J. 1981. Failure to identify venereal disease in a lesbian population. *Sexually Transmitted Diseases* 8(2):75–76.

Rossi PH, Wright JD, Fisher GA, Willis G. 1987. The urban homeless: Estimating composition and size. Science 235:1336–1341.

Russell JM, Azadian BS, Roberts AP, Talboys CA. 1995. Pharyngeal flora in a sexually active population. *International Journal of STD and AIDS* 6(3):211–215.

Sell RL, Petrulio C. 1996. Sampling homosexuals, bisexuals, gays, and lesbians for public health research: A review of the literature from 1990 to 1992. *Journal of Homosexuality* 30(4):31–47.

Shaffer D, Fisher P, Hicks RH, Parides M, Gould M. 1995. Sexual orientation in adolescents who commit suicide. *Suicide and Life-Threatening Behavior* 25(Suppl):64–71.

Smith EM, Johnson SR, Guenther SM. 1985. Health care attitudes and experiences during gynecologic care among lesbians and bisexuals. *American Journal of Public Health* 75(9):1085–1087.

Trevathan WR, Burleson MH, Gregory WL. 1993. No evidence for menstrual synchrony in lesbian couples. *Psychoneuroendocrinology* 18(5–6):425–435.

Trippet SE. 1994. Lesbians' mental health concerns. *Health Care for Women International* 15(4):317–323.

Turner CF. 1997. Presentation before the Institute of Medicine Committee on Lesbian Health Research Priorities. Washington, DC, October 6–7, 1997.

Turner CF, Forsyth BH, O'Reilly J, Cooley PC, Smith TK, Rogers SM, Miller HG. 1998a. Automated self-interviewing and the survey measurement of sensitive behaviors. In: Couper M, et al., eds. *Computer-Assisted Survey Information Collection*. New York: Wiley and Sons.

Turner CF, Ku L, Rogers SM, Lindberg LD, Pleck JH, Sonenstein FL. 1998b. Adolescent sexual behavior, drug use, and violence: Increased reporting with computer survey technology. *Science* 280:867–873.

Turner CF, Lessler JT, Devore J. 1992. Effects of mode administration and wording on reporting of drug use. In: Turner CF, Lessler JT, Gfroerer JD, eds. *Survey Measurement of Drug Use: Methodological Issues*. DHHS Pub. No. 92-1929. Washington, DC: U.S. Government Printing Office.

Women's Health Initiative Study Group. 1998. Design of the Women's Health Initiative Clinical Trial and Observational Study. *Controlled Clinical Trials* 19:61–109.

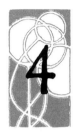

Contextual Barriers to Conducting Research on Lesbian Health

As in many areas of health research, the investigation of lesbian health operates in a context of factors such as political pressures (both national and research institution based), funding availability, and community attitudes. For researchers focusing on lesbian health, however, some of these pressures present particularly challenging obstacles. In this section, some of the contextual barriers to conducting research on lesbian health are reviewed, including the political context, the importance of establishing connections between researchers and the lesbian community, and the difficulties encountered by those wishing to conduct research on lesbian health.

BARRIERS TO CONDUCTING RESEARCH

For numerous reasons, researchers in academic and other settings (e.g., independent research institutes, clinical research centers, community research organizations) have been reluctant to initiate research on lesbian health. Many of the historical barriers continue to affect what research is done, how it is perceived, what kinds of resources are made available, and the personal and professional impact on those who conduct lesbian research.

The committee identified several factors that have acted to inhibit the conduct of research on lesbians. As has already been noted, some of the reluctance to conduct research in this area arises because of the difficult methodological challenges that researchers face in designing and implementing sound studies of lesbians (e.g., because lesbians have been a hidden population, finding a diverse and representative sample can be extremely difficult). There are numerous other barriers, including the potential negative effects on academic careers of working with a stigmatized population, the lack of mentors for conducting research in this area, and the lack of funding.

Potential Negative Career Ramifications Due to Stigma[1]

A woman researcher's lesbian sexual orientation can have a negative impact on her work experience in two primary ways. First, if she conducts lesbian-related research, her career may be negatively affected because of stigma associated with the lesbian population. Second, she may experience negative effects, such as discrimination, because she herself is lesbian, a problem potentially experienced by lesbians no matter what their work setting. Very few research organizations provide an environment in which lesbian researchers can (1) reveal their lesbian sexual orientation to colleagues and students without experiencing negative consequences, and (2) pursue research about lesbians without negative repercussions (Ryan and Bradford, 1997). In a survey by Ryan and Bradford (1997) of 284 lesbian researchers from 41 states and 14 countries, more than half of whom had been working as researchers for 10 or more years, both negative and positive experiences were reported as a result of being a lesbian and conducting research about lesbians. Of the lesbian researchers surveyed, 30% reported that they specialized in lesbian-related research. More negative career sanctions were associated with being a lesbian, however, than with conducting lesbian-related research.

---

[1]The following sections incorporate significant portions of the workshop presentation by Caitlin Ryan.

Stigma Associated with Conducting Lesbian Research

Fear of negative career repercussions has prevented some lesbian and non-lesbian researchers, particularly in academic settings, from conducting lesbian-related research. The demands of attaining tenure in academia and promotions in nonacademic research organizations are so arduous that researchers interested in studying lesbians may feel they have to choose between research in this area and the pursuit of professional success. Most of the gay and lesbian academics surveyed by McNaron (1997) acknowledged that significant gains had been made, but many still felt that research on lesbian or gay issues was professionally risky. Although the committee is unaware of research in this area, it is reasonable to expect that similar pressures deter researchers in nonacademic research institutes and clinical settings from pursuing research on lesbian issues.

Of the lesbian researchers surveyed by Ryan and Bradford (1997), less than one-third (29%) reported having a very supportive environment for conducting research on lesbian issues. Almost a quarter (23%) reported that conducting lesbian-related research had a somewhat or very negative impact on finding a mentor, adviser, or consultant; 26% reported negative impact on obtaining grant funding; and 23% reported negative impact on finding a job. Finally, a survey of graduate student members of the American Psychological Association Division 44, the division for the study of lesbian, gay, and bisexual issues, found that more than half of the students surveyed reported negative experiences from conducting research in this area (Pilkington and Cantor, 1996). The negative experiences included exposure to antigay or biased textbooks and course materials, offensive and biased comments from instructors, and a range of negative and discriminatory experiences with faculty, administrative staff, and interns. Approximately one out of three students was discouraged or warned that research on sexual orientation would have negative career consequences, or had experienced specific interference or refusal to allow research on lesbian and gay issues.

Stigma Associated with Being a Lesbian in Research Settings

The few studies on experiences that lesbian or gay researchers have with bias and discrimination have found significant levels of professional bias and negative career consequences. In surveys of gay, lesbian, and bisexual members of the American Sociological Association in 1981 and 1992 (Gagnon et al., 1982; Taylor and Raebrun, 1995), researchers who were open at work about their sexual orientation reported more experiences of bias related to their sexual orientation than those who were not. Such bias included discrimination in hiring, tenure, promotion, and scholarly devaluation; exclusion from social and professional networks; harassment and intimidation.

McNaron (1997) studied gay and lesbian academics with more than 15 years of teaching and research experience. Most reported that although their institutions had antidiscrimination policies in place, they felt that their sexual orientation had an impact on their work experience. Only half of the academics had come out to department chairs and administrators, and about a third were open to their students. Approximately one out of four of the lesbian researchers surveyed by Ryan and Bradford (1997) reported believing that their difficulty in finding or keeping a job or in getting a promotion or obtaining tenure was due to being lesbian. Because no comparison group was included, however, it is not possible to determine how these experiences compare to those of other researchers.

Isolation of Lesbians in Research Settings and Lack of Academic Mentors

The limited number of people conducting research on lesbian issues has implications both for lesbian researchers and for students interesting in pursuing careers conducting research on lesbian issues. Lack of access to colleagues, mentors, and other researchers who are lesbian was cited as a major barrier to personal and professional development for the lesbian researchers surveyed by Ryan and Bradford (1997). Nine out of ten respondents ranked access to lesbian researchers as their top priority, and three-quarters said that mentoring was their primary need.

Students who wish to pursue research careers that focus on lesbian issues face several challenges stemming from the lack of access to mentors who conduct research with lesbians. In a recent study of the experiences that lesbian psychology students have in conducting lesbian research, students reported difficulty finding supportive mentors, research advisers, or dissertation committee members; being required to educate advisers about lesbian issues; a lack of peer support; a lack of necessary materials in the university library; being held to a higher standard than other students; and concerns about getting their research published (Morris, 1995). Given these difficulties, students who might pursue research careers in lesbian health may themselves, or through the efforts of peers and colleagues, be directed to other areas of research study, thus reducing the pool of future researchers in lesbian health issues.

Lack of Funding to Study Lesbian Health

The lack of funding to support research on lesbian health hampered early efforts of researchers to conduct studies and has slowed the follow-up on specific findings. Lesbian health research has been criticized for lacking scientific rigor usually because of its use of non-probability samples and the lack of appropriate comparison groups. At the same time, with money in short supply for this area of research, it has been difficult to design and implement methodologically rigorous studies, which require larger budgets. The difficulty in obtaining funds is felt acutely by researchers doing clinical projects. Randomized, controlled clinical trials—the gold standard in clinical intervention research—do not now play a significant role in lesbian health research—the exception being the Women's Health Initiative (WHI), which includes some lesbian participants. The committee believes, however, that randomized clinical trials with lesbians are probably premature at this time because of the lack of evidence indicating differential health problems in lesbians.[2]

There are few sources for funding clinical research about lesbians. Although some foundations, including the Lesbian Health Fund of the Gay and Lesbian Medical Association, have begun to support studies in this area, the amounts are generally too small (typically around $7,000, the maximum amount available per grant) for substantial efforts. Major foundations have provided limited funds for lesbian, gay, and bisexual research outside the AIDS arena, and competition is high for the more limited

[2]An exception might be a trial on health care utilization by lesbians.

lesbian and gay funding sources. It is important to note that some federal funding for lesbian health research has been provided in recent years, notably through administrative supplements made available through the National Institutes of Health (NIH) Office of Research on Women's Health and initiatives supported by the Centers for Disease Control and Prevention (CDC) (see Table 4.1 and Box 4.1, respectively). Some funding has also been made available from the National Institute on Drug Abuse (NIDA),[3] the National Institute of Mental Health (NIMH),[4] and the National Institute of Allergy and Infectious Diseases (NIAID).[5]

The majority of research on lesbian health conducted to date has come from within the lesbian community itself, most of it with little funding and very few resources. Smaller pilot projects have often been done on a shoestring budget or have been added onto other funded projects without supplemental funding to cover the additional costs associated with data collection and analyses. The difficulty in obtaining funding, even for pilot studies, subsequently affects researchers' ability to compile the data needed to apply successfully for federal research dollars.

Difficulties in Publishing Research and Disseminating Findings

There is a growing body of published information on lesbian health, which is summarized in Appendix A. Nonetheless, much research from community-based or initiated studies is not published in the scientific literature, and academic studies usually are not shared outside the professional literature. There are likely numerous reasons why more published research on lesbian health does not appear in scientific journals. In some cases, this may be because the work lacks scientific rigor. Researchers on lesbian health report finding it difficult to publish the results of their work. Data are not available, however, to determine the specific nature of the barriers to publishing lesbian-related research. For example, it is not known

[3]NIDA has funded a study to examine HIV risk among women injection drug users who have sex with women.
[4]Studies funded by NIMH include research on HIV risk and coming out among gay and lesbian adolescents and on the mental health consequences of antigay and antilesbian violence.
[5]NIAID has funded a study that includes a component examining the transmission of genital herpes simplex virus between herpes-discordant lesbian partners.

TABLE 4.1 Lesbian Health Grant Supplements Funded by NIH Through the National Cancer Institute Interagency Agreement

Grant Title	Study Goals	Funded Institution
Improving Adherence in Women at Risk for Breast Cancer	Investigate barriers to breast cancer screening faced by women at high risk. Supplemental funding used to collect data from 200 lesbians. Project will develop and pilot-test a breast cancer risk counseling intervention tailored to the unique needs of lesbians at increased risk for breast cancer.	Georgetown University
Increasing Breast Screening Among Nonadherent Women	Identify the knowledge, beliefs, and practices of lesbians regarding breast cancer specifically and health promotion more generally; evaluate the risk factors for lesbians; and develop and test culturally competent health education interventions.	Duke University
A Multicenter Trial of Group Therapy for Breast Cancer Patients	Assess and compare lesbian and heterosexual women's psychosocial adjustment to breast cancer; examine the usefulness of supportive or expressive group psychotherapy for lesbians with breast cancer.	Stanford University
Adjustment to Breast Cancer Among Younger Women	Explore factors that contribute to distress of young breast cancer patients during diagnosis and treatment; test a counseling intervention to address issues of vulnerability and resilience that affect psychosocial outlook. Supplement used to replicate the study in an ethnically diverse cohort of lesbian breast cancer patients.	Miami University
Nursing Strategies to Promote Breast Cancer Screening	Determine the effects of theory-based informational messages delivered by nurses on use of breast cancer screening among women who have not had mammography as recommended; examine whether the effects of messages on breast cancer screening rates are associated with sexual orientation.	University of Wisconsin

BOX 4.1
CDC Research and Programs That Include Lesbians, 1997

The CDC has a number of research and other initiatives that include a focus on lesbians. These activities include the following:

National Breast and Cervical Cancer Early Detection Program

• Outreach efforts are piloted through funding four demonstration projects with the Young Women's Christian Association (YWCA) of the United States (U.S.) and ENCOREplus programs.
• A partnership between the YWCA and the Mautner Project for Lesbians with Cancer was established to design and test specific outreach strategies for breast and cervical cancer screening for older lesbians in four sites across the country.

HIV/AIDS

• Lesbians are recognized as a population of interest in which to address risks of HIV. Efforts are directed toward research into behavioral risk factors and toward quantifying risks of women who have sex with women, as well as the prevention needs of this population.
• The HIV Epidemiology Research Study, a multicenter women's HIV cohort study, addresses issues related to HIV and lesbians.
• Funding (FY 1997) for a woman-to-woman HIV transmission study has been awarded that will be carried out in four sites: (1) Yale University; (2) the Lyon-Martin Center in San Francisco; (3) the Lesbian AIDS Project in New York City; and (4) the Whitman-Walker Clinic in Washington, D.C.
• In April 1995, the CDC carried out an external consultation to review the science on woman-to-woman transmission of HIV and to look at prevention needs of lesbians.

Violence

The National Center for Injury Prevention and Control convened a workshop in 1994 to develop recommendations for a research agenda in suicide and sexual orientation. These recommendations were published in a fall 1995 supplement to the journal *Suicide and Life-Threatening Behavior*.

SOURCE: Jones, 1997.

how many articles are actually submitted each year or the acceptance and rejection rates of papers on lesbian health. During the workshop the committee heard anecdotal statements that some journal editors and reviewers are reluctant to publish such work or to believe that it may be of interest to a broader audience. However, additional empirical information is needed before clear conclusions can be drawn regarding the factors that impede publication of lesbian-related research articles.

> *I once had a manuscript returned to me unreviewed by a top journal, the only time in my career this has ever happened, because the editor informed me that his readers were not interested in research on black lesbians. He implied that the sample must be biased, because it was difficult to imagine that my research team could find 600 black lesbians to fill out the questionnaires in the first place.*
>
> Susan Cochran, Public Workshop, October 6–7, 1997
> Washington, D.C.

The committee notes that a number of articles on lesbian health topics have been published in major biomedical journals (see Appendix A).[6] The committee believes, however, that the importance of research on lesbian health is such that it is desirable that more research on this topic be published in mainstream biomedical and behavioral health journals. In addition to being relevant to issues of women's health in general, this research is more broadly applicable or of interest to those conducting research on other sensitive behaviors or hard-to-reach populations; those interested in issues of cultural diversity and the impact of stress on health or resiliency; and so forth. The committee urges journal editors and reviewers to take this into account in reaching decisions about which high-quality papers should be accepted for publication.

---

[6]An important development for the field of lesbian health is that the Gay and Lesbian Medical Association recently began publication of a journal that deals exclusively with lesbian and gay health issues, the *Journal of the Gay and Lesbian Medical Association.*

Researchers are not surprised to have received rejection letters that say "thank you for this manuscript, but we have already published one paper on lesbian health this year," or "thank you for this manuscript but lesbian health is not important to our readers."

Jocelyn White, Public Workshop, October 6–7, 1997
Washington, D.C.

Strategies to Provide a Supportive Lesbian Health Research Infrastructure

There are a number of promising strategies that would enhance the ability of researchers to conduct research on lesbian health. The committee urges the NIH, including the Office of Research on Women's Health, to identify mechanisms for initiating these strategies in collaboration with representatives of the lesbian health community:

• Develop communication and information-sharing system(s) for lesbian health research issues and resources (e.g., information clearinghouses, web pages, and e-mail-based discussion lists) focused on discussion and dissemination of information on lesbian health research.
• Formalize a network of mentors at universities, independent research institutes, clinical research sites, and training centers throughout the country to provide mentoring support to students and peer support for researchers and academics interested in conducting such research.
• Offer technical assistance and training to those interested in conducting research on lesbian health to enable them to deal with the complex methodological challenges involved in designing and implementing these studies, including forming and managing collaborative research teams that include active participation from members of the study population.

Further, the committee urges that the availability of federal funding be increased to support additional research on lesbian health and that funding mechanisms be developed to support doctoral and postdoctoral training in lesbian health research.

THE NEED FOR RESEARCHER–COMMUNITY TIES[7]

The community–researcher link is a very important part of lesbian health research, as it is for other research that involves hard-to-identify, stigmatized, or culturally distinct groups.[8] This link stimulates the development of important research questions, facilitates participation by research subjects, keeps researchers informed of important activities and changes in the research population, and provides opportunities for feedback to research participants. Researcher–community collaboration is critical for increasing the understanding of lesbians and their health needs. Historically, much research on lesbians has been conducted by community-based researchers and by master's and doctoral students, often lesbians themselves. This trend continues today, and important research on lesbians continues to be stimulated and carried out in community-based settings.

When working with hard-to-reach populations and populations with specific needs, it is especially important to gain the perspectives of those who have a stake in the research, particularly members of the population of concern. This input can be solicited in a variety of ways. For example, focus groups can be assembled to review the need for the research, research questions, research plans, protocols and measurements, and outcomes of importance.[9] Involving the community in the process of designing a study can produce a number of important benefits. A cooperative partnership between researchers and the community can help ensure that the research is feasible and that the fidelity of a study design is maintained. For example, staff at a community organization may have important insights into the types of people who use their services, what kinds of interventions could be promising, what procedures in an experimental protocol might be particularly difficult to implement, how to approach

---

[7]This section incorporate portions of the workshop presentations by Joyce Hunter and Debra Rog.

[8]By "community," the committee means a group of people, not necessarily living in the same geographic neighborhood, who are drawn together because of shared interests, values, or characteristics and who share or develop resources that address their interests. Thus, in this case, the lesbian community would include the network of resources and activities focused on the interests of lesbians in a particular area.

[9]Community advisory committees have been used widely and successfully in HIV/AIDS research to accomplish this task.

potential study participants in a way that is likely to result in participation, and so forth. Getting this kind of community-level feedback can be essential for the success of a research study.

Commonly, lesbian researchers who conduct research on lesbian health already have deep and active ties to the lesbian community. Thus, they come with an indigenous understanding of the concerns of the community, at least for the subgroups of lesbians with which they are most closely affiliated (e.g., those involved in lesbian organizations or activities). However, this knowledge does *not* ensure understanding of the particular population under study, which may differ in terms of class, race and ethnicity, age, and so forth. Researchers who do not know the community must be willing to take the time and effort to learn about it. Because stereotypes about lesbian life are so pervasive and lesbians are not an especially visible community, there is a danger that researchers who do not familiarize themselves with the concerns of lesbians will choose to study topics that the community may not find useful or will misinterpret or misunderstand the implications of their results. If this happens, the willingness of the community to provide information freely will understandably be compromised. Lesbian, gay, and bisexual populations are, for the most part, marginalized. They may be suspicious of researchers and resistant to observation; this may be particularly true in lesbian and gay communities of color.

There are numerous ways in which both the researcher and the community stand to benefit from researcher–community collaboration.

Potential benefits for the researcher include the following:

• getting support for and cooperation with the research;
• helping to avoid bias;
• gaining an understanding of participants' concerns and fears, special needs, and disincentives to participate;
• ensuring that the right questions are asked;
• facilitating the participation of subjects;
• increasing the understanding of results;
• helping to develop ideas and analytic directions; and
• ensuring that the study design is feasible in a particular setting.

Potential benefits to the community include

- methodologic expertise necessary to ensure meaningful, quality studies;
- data to help justify funding for health care and education programs;
- information on potentially modifiable risk factors;
- high-quality research that leads to a better understanding of lesbian health issues; and
- opportunity to pilot-test models for service provision.

I just can't emphasize that too strongly, how important it was to get and recruit and train good people to go out and get lesbians in communities where the university-based researchers do not have some natural allegiance.

Ann Pollinger Haas, Public Workshop, October 6–7, 1997
Washington, D.C.

Researchers, community members, and community organizations have expertise, although usually in different areas. Factors that can influence the success of researcher–community partnerships include the following:

- **Prior establishment of trust and a working relationship between the lesbian community and the researchers.**
- **Belief in the outcome of the research.** Organizations in communities where research is being conducted will want to know what impact the research study will have on their clients and their organization. This can be facilitated by involving community members and organizations in the development of the research intervention.
- **Involvement from the ground up in the development of the program.** The participation of community organizations in the development of research interventions will help ensure that the research

does not disrupt or interfere with their ongoing programs. It is important that community organizations not be presented with a finished product that is difficult to adopt or retrofit into their existing programs. It is important to have input and involvement of the source population in the interpretation and reporting of data, as well as during the design of the research.

• **An understanding of limitations of resources and of different priorities.** It may be important to reimburse community organizations for the time lost by personnel because of participation in the research. Such reimbursements not only establish trust and goodwill but also compensate for loss of staff time available to accomplish the activities of the community organization.

• **Researchers "give back" to the community.** Communities are often not informed of the results of research studies in which they have been involved. Stakeholders can and should be involved in the discussion of how research results can be used to improve the health of lesbians.

• **Concerns about how confidentiality of information, particularly about sexual orientation, will be maintained must be addressed to the satisfaction of community-based agencies and potential research participants.**

POLITICAL AND LEGISLATIVE BARRIERS TO FUNDING

Research on controversial or sensitive topics, such as sexual behavior, sexual orientation, or drug use, can quickly become embroiled in politics. Researchers interested in doing wide-scale studies of sexual behaviors have faced numerous political challenges to the conduct of research in this area. In fact, it has taken the AIDS crisis to begin to alleviate the historical dearth of federally funded survey research examining the range of sexual behaviors in the United States (NRC, 1989; Laumann et al., 1994a).

The experience of the National Opinion Research Center (NORC) in Chicago in conducting its national survey of sexual behavior provides an informative example of the effects of political pressures on the accomplishment of such research, particularly when data might be gathered on same-sex sexual behavior. In 1987, the National Institute of Child Health and Human Development (NICHD) issued a request for proposals to design a national survey of adult sexual behaviors, which was subsequently awarded to the NORC (Laumann et al., 1994a,b). The study included as its goals the collection of information about human sexuality, as well as information relevant to intervention programs for sexually transmitted infections, such as HIV. Subsequently, the study group was awarded a contract to begin the collection of data to demonstrate the feasibility of a larger national survey. The survey instrument was modified numerous times as the researchers and NICHD worked to develop an instrument that would be acceptable to the Office of Management and Budget, which must approve surveys designed under federal contract, and the Department of Health and Human Services (DHHS). In doing so, focus on the collection of basic data on human sexuality was minimized in an effort to secure approval. Nonetheless, even a more narrowly focused interview instrument failed to obtain approval during the four years of the next administration. Additionally, Congress failed to authorize funding for the study during this period, with some members of Congress being vociferous opponents of the study. Ultimately, after it became clear in 1991 that strong opposition to the study by key members of Congress would make it very difficult for NICHD to provide funding for the survey, the NORC research team decided to forgo federal support and secured funding from a consortium of private foundations to conduct its comprehensive national study of sexual behavior.

A national study on adolescent sexuality faced similar opposition from some members of Congress, particularly Jesse Helms (R–NC) (Laumann et al., 1994b; *Time*, 1991).[10] Eventually researchers at the University of North Carolina were able to go forward with a related study despite federal concerns and reluctance to fund it.

At the workshop, several possible political responses were identified that can have potentially negative consequences on the future of research on lesbian health (Gostin, 1997). For example, it was suggested that legis-

---

[10]Senator Helms offered the following amendment to the National Institutes of Health Revitalization Act, 1992: "The Secretary of Health and Human Services may not during fiscal year 1992 or any subsequent fiscal year conduct or support the SHARP [Survey of Health and AIDS Risk Prevalence] survey of adult sexual behavior or the American Teenage Study of adolescent sexual behavior." This amendment was adopted by the Senate, 51 to 46 (*Congressional Record*, April 2, 1991).

lators might deny the existence of lesbians or, as is more likely, not recognize that their health issues are legitimate areas for broader concern. Another possible political response is to classify a particular behavior or identity as immoral. A belief that a behavior is immoral and a perception that a research or policy response somehow encourages this immoral behavior can impede research. It may be viewed as a less legitimate topic for federal research funding due to the perceived immorality. The research itself may be viewed as immoral, or more realistically, the research may somehow be considered to legitimize the behavior. Finally, another possible political response is to classify the status of being lesbian, or same-sex behavior, as unhealthy or a risk factor in and of itself, with resulting implications for funding lesbian health initiatives. This response can, moreover, potentially lead to discrimination against the group (e.g., differential health insurance costs even if individuals do not carry higher levels of scientifically identified risk).

ETHICAL CONSIDERATIONS[11]

Given the limitations and scope of this workshop study the committee was unable to consider in depth the ethical issues related to the conduct of research on lesbian health.

Nonetheless, the committee believes these issues to be of very great importance and so highlights here some of the concerns discussed at the workshop pertaining to the potential risks involved in participating in research and to the confidentiality of data.[12]

---

[11]This section is based largely on the workshop presentation by Larry Norton.

[12]More in-depth discussions of the ethical issues involved in conducting research with stigmatized populations, or involving the collection of data on stigmatized, sensitive, or illegal behaviors, are available. For example, the National Research Council (NRC) Committee on AIDS Research and the Behavioral, Social, and Statistical Sciences (NRC, 1989) considered issues of confidentiality in collecting information on sensitive behaviors, and the report of the NRC Committee on Evaluating Genetic Diversity (NRC, 1997) provides more detailed discussion of issues of privacy and consent related to the storage and future use of tissue samples. Laumann et al. (1994a) also consider issues of confidentiality and privacy in the context of their national study of sexual behavior. Boruch and Cecil (1979) provide a general reference on ensuring the confidentiality of social research data.

The reader is also advised to look to research with other populations as a potentially helpful strategy for informing research on lesbian health. These include, for example, research with gay men (who share some of the same concerns regarding disclosure), research on minority populations (who similarly experience discrimination), and research on women in general.

Risks to Research Participants

Participating in research carries potential risks for lesbians, both as individual research participants and as members of a particular population group. As individuals, for example, participating in research can increase the chances that one's lesbian sexual orientation will be disclosed to others (e.g., through the sharing of databases if the data include identifiers). If the research participant has previously chosen not to disclose her sexual orientation publicly, perceived risks of disclosure can present a disincentive to participating in the research.

Of greater concern are the risks that research on lesbians may have to the population of lesbians as a whole, particularly given the pervasiveness of societal homophobia. This includes the risk that research information will be used in some way to discriminate against or stigmatize lesbians in general. For example, if lesbians as a group were found to be at higher risk for a particular health problem, providers of health or life insurance might argue that they should be denied coverage or charged higher premiums, because their increased likelihood of incurring higher health costs or having a shorter life span increases the risk for insurers. Another potential risk relates to the privacy concerns of the social groups of lesbians to which individuals belong (Laumann et al., 1994a). Even when individuals give informed consent to participate in research, in the process of responding they may reveal information that violates the privacy of their sexual partners, as well as the privacy of the group. Although the committee acknowledges these potential risks, the committee also believes that significant benefits to the lesbian population can accrue from studying lesbian health, provided careful protection of individual rights is in place. These include identifying areas of increased risk that need attention, identifying gaps in services, and increasing understanding of the negative impact of homophobia on health.

In the case of the participation of gay men in studies of AIDS, barriers to participation were overcome by a sense of community that emerged from the feeling that this is a problem faced by all members of the gay community. To what extent organized lesbian groups will strongly advocate a research agenda is yet to be determined and may vary depending on the focus of the research and the ways in which community involvement is sought.

Confidentiality

Maintaining confidentiality is a key concern in studies with lesbians. Information collected from an individual can be regarded as confidential with respect to others if it will not be disclosed to anyone else in an identifiable manner without the specific consent of the individual who supplied the information   (Boruch and Cecil, 1979; Laumann et al., 1994a). Because being lesbian is often stigmatized and some same-sex behaviors are illegal in some jurisdictions, concerns are heightened about how information gathered about sexual orientation will be used (Platzer and James, 1997).

Numerous strategies can be employed to ensure confidentiality, such as using coded identifiers instead of names (Boruch and Cecil, 1979). However, although keeping data completely anonymous clearly protects confidentiality, it also precludes follow-up of nonrespondents and accurate calculation of response rates, as well as the longitudinal follow-up of respondents to assess changes over time. Strategies that ensure confidentiality help to secure research participation and elicit candid responses only to the extent respondents actually *believe* that the information gathered will be kept confidential.

Certain, but not all, public databases are shared among groups such as health care providers, government organizations, and public health departments. Often these data files are linked to unique identifiers, such as a social security number. This is true for many large-scale government surveys where information is used to link sources of data and to help in locating people in order to collect longitudinal data. At the workshop, several participants expressed concerns about gathering information on sexual orientation in government surveys, with some voicing fears that information gathered in one survey might be used as a way to identify lesbians for some harmful purpose (e.g., to detect illegal behavior, to limit access to services). Whether or not these fears are well founded, they illustrate some of the heightened sensitivity regarding confidentiality.

Reliable data are not available on the degree to which lesbians are trustful of researchers, particularly in cases of government surveys, although it is likely that concerns regarding confidentiality have an impact on both their level of participation in these surveys and how candid they are in their responses. The committee concludes that research is needed on whether lesbians will answer sensitive questions about their sexual orientation and health-related practices on confidential government surveys that have personal identifiers.

Several additional issues were brought up during the workshop about which the committee urges further discussion among researchers, lesbians, and funders:

- What are the specific questions that institutional review boards[13] should consider when evaluating research involving lesbians, and are there particular directions or instructions that should be provided to institutional review boards to aid them in evaluating research involving lesbians, particularly with respect to confidentiality?
- What considerations are unique to obtaining informed consent from participants in research on lesbian health, including consideration of the potential risks and benefits of participation? What considerations should be given to obtaining consent for minors to participate in research where information on same-sex behaviors will be gathered, especially given that parents may not be aware of their child's sexual orientation?
- What procedures are most effective for ensuring that confidentiality is maintained in research with lesbians?[14] Is there a need to develop new mechanisms?
- What unique issues are involved in the future use of data collected from lesbians, including the collection of genetic information?
- What is the range of privacy issues involved in conducting research on lesbian health, and are there special considerations that should be given to protecting the privacy of both individual research participants and the larger population of lesbians?

---

[13]Institutional review boards are responsible for reviewing research proposals to ensure that they are in compliance with institutional and federal regulations regarding the protection of human subjects. Institutional review board approval is required for federally funded research involving human subjects.

[14]Under federal law, researchers can obtain a Certificate of Confidentiality to protect research data from being disclosed under subpoena. The types of information that may be protected by a Certificate of Confidentiality include drug use, alcohol use, illegal behavior or activities or sexual practices or preferences.

REFERENCES

Boruch RF, Cecil JS. 1979. *Assuring the Confidentiality of Social Research Data.* Philadelphia: University of Pennsylvania Press.

Gagnon JH, Rosen RC, Leiblum SR. 1982. Cognitive and social aspects of sexual dysfunction: Sexual scripts in sex therapy. *Journal of Sex and Marital Therapy* 8(1):44–56.

Gostin L. 1997. "Ethical Issues in Conducting Research with Lesbians." Presentation at the Institute of Medicine Workshop on Lesbian Health Research Priorities. Washington, DC: October 6–7, 1997.

Jones WK. 1997. Personal communication, September 19. Washington, DC: Centers for Disease Control and Prevention.

Laumann EO, Gagnon JH, Michael RT, Michaels S. 1994a. *The Social Organization of Sexuality: Sexual Practices in the United States.* Chicago: University of Chicago Press.

Laumann EO, Michael RT, Gagnon JH. 1994b. A political history of the national sex survey of adults. *Family Planning Perspectives* 26(1):34–38.

McNaron TAH. 1997. *Poisoned Ivy: Lesbian and Gay Academics Confronting Homophobia.* Philadelphia: Temple University Press.

Morris JF. 1995. *A Graduate Student Perspective on Issues in Lesbian Research.* Paper presented at the American Psychological Association Conference, New York, August 1995.

NRC (National Research Council). 1989. *AIDS: Sexual Behavior and Intravenous Drug Use.* Washington, DC: National Academy Press.

NRC. 1997. *Evaluating Genetic Diversity.* Washington, DC: National Academy Press.

Pilkington NW, Cantor JM. 1996. Perceptions of heterosexual bias in professional psychology programs: A survey of graduate students. *Professional Psychology: Research and Practice* 27(6):604–612.

Platzer H, James T. 1997. Methodological issues conducting sensitive research on lesbian and gay men's experience of nursing care. *Journal of Advanced Nursing* 25(3):626–633.

Ryan C, Bradford J. 1997. *Lesbian Research Network: Final Report—Year 1.* Richmond, VA: An Uncommon Legacy Foundation.

Taylor V, Raebrun N. 1995. Identity politics as high-risk activism: Career consequences for lesbian, gay and bisexual sociologists. Social Problems 42(2):252–273.

Time. 1991. No sex, we're Republicans. *Time* August 5:27.

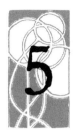

Conclusions and Recommendations

The following conclusions, recommendations, and research priorities are based on the workshop presentations, the testimony submitted to the committee, a review of the relevant literature, and the committee's discussion of the issues. The key points underlying the recommendations and research priorities are outlined here; more detailed supporting information can be found in the preceding chapters.

CONCLUSIONS

The committee reached three major conclusions:

Conclusion 1: Additional data are required to determine if lesbians may be at higher risk for certain health problems. Further research is needed to determine the absolute and relative magnitudes of such risk and to better understand the risk and protective factors that influence lesbian health.

Conclusion 2: There are significant barriers to conducting research on lesbian health, including lack of funding, which have limited the development of more sophisticated studies, data analyses, and the publication of results.

Conclusion 3: Research on lesbian health, especially the development of more sophisticated methodologies to conduct such research, will help advance scientific knowledge that is also of benefit to other population subgroups, including rare or hard-to-identify population subgroups and women in general.

The committee identified numerous areas where additional research is needed either to better understand lesbian health or to improve the methods used to study lesbians and their health. Priority areas for research are the following:

Research Priority 1: Research is needed to better understand the physical and mental health status of lesbians and to determine whether there are health problems for which lesbians are at higher risk as well as conditions for which protective factors operate to reduce their health risk.

There has been much speculation about health risks of lesbians, and there is some evidence that lesbians may be at heightened risk for some problems. There are, however, large data gaps in the knowledge about lesbian health, and the population-based data needed to determine the relative health risks of this population are not available. It is critical that such research consider the socioeconomic and cultural contexts in which lesbians live and the impact of these factors on their health. Risk factors that influence the health of lesbians across the life span include negative attitudes and stigma toward them, barriers in access to health care, socio-economic factors, various legal factors including the fact that engaging in lesbian sexual behavior is illegal in some states, and the stresses associated with all of these factors. However, little is known about the specific impact of these risk factors on lesbian health and even less about any unique protective factors and how they may operate.

Research Priority 2: Research is needed to better understand how to define sexual orientation in general and lesbian sexual orientation in particular and to better understand the diversity of the lesbian population.

Definitions of lesbian samples in research studies have varied widely along the multiple dimensions of sexual orientation: sexual identity, sexual behavior, and attraction or desire. Only in some cases are definitions conceptualized based on the goals of a particular study. Population-based data are needed to better understand these dimensions of sexual orientation and the interrelationships among them.

Lesbians are a very diverse group, varying along dimensions of sexual orientation and in terms of demographic characteristics such as socioeconomic status, race and ethnicity, culture, religious background, and age. Population-based "baseline" studies are needed to better understand the characteristics of the population and how these characteristics interrelate with health status. Studies are especially needed to better understand the developmental course of lesbians across the life span. In particular, research is needed on the impact of stigma on lesbians across the life span, especially among different racial and ethnic groups and a range of socioeconomic classes. International and cross-cultural studies may also be helpful for increasing understanding of the interrelationships among these factors and their impact on lesbian health. Because the field of lesbian health research is still relatively undeveloped, studies are needed that use qualitative research methods, such as ethnographies and focus groups, to increase understanding of the diversity and distinct subgroupings and behaviors of the population.

Research Priority 3: Research is needed to identify possible barriers to access to mental and physical health care services for lesbians and ways to increase their access to these services.

It is commonly believed in the lesbian community that lesbians fail to access traditional health services at the same levels as other women, although population-based data are not available to determine the degree to which this problem exists. Nonetheless, the committee did identify a number of barriers to access to mental and physical health care services for lesbians. These include structural barriers, such as the potential impact of managed care and the lack of legal recognition of relationship partners; financial barriers, which have an impact on access to health insurance coverage; and personal and cultural barriers, including attitudes of health care providers and the lack of cultural competency among providers for addressing the needs of lesbian clients. Increased understanding of the barriers to health care for lesbians can provide useful information for understanding and improving access for other underserved groups as well.

In addition to the general conclusions and research priorities, the committee makes eight recommendations for improving the knowledge base on lesbian health.

RECOMMENDATIONS

Recommendation 1: Public and private funding to support research on lesbian health needs to be increased in order to enhance knowledge about risks to health and protective factors, to improve methodologies for gathering information about lesbian health, to increase understanding of the diversity of the lesbian population, and to improve lesbians' access to mental and physical health care services.

A long-term federal funding commitment to lesbian health research is needed that is responsive to the ongoing needs of the lesbian population. Foundations and other government entities are also urged to fund research on lesbian health.

Recommendation 2: Methodological research needs to be funded and conducted to improve measurement of the various dimensions of lesbian sexual orientation.

Methodological research is needed to improve and refine the methods available to study lesbian health. The committee recommends that methodological research be funded and conducted to improve measurement of the various dimensions of lesbian orientation: identity, behavior, and attraction, including women of different racial and ethnic groups, social classes, ages and birth cohorts, religious backgrounds, and geographical areas. Although existing questions on surveys are adequate for many research purposes, further work is needed to assess and improve their validity. Methodological research is also needed on the feasibility of using different sampling techniques, by themselves or in combination, for rare or hard-to-identify populations, to obtain a probability sample of the lesbian population.

Funding is also needed for start-up studies on lesbian health, supplements to ongoing studies to include and analyze responses to questions regarding lesbian health, secondary analyses of existing data, and conferences focusing on methodological and ethical issues in lesbian health research.

Furthermore, the committee takes note of the fact that a disproportionate amount of work in this area has focused on lesbians with ties to lesbian community organizations and events. An unknown, but possibly sizable, number of lesbians do not have such ties to organizations and so are routinely missed in such studies. Thus, research is needed to determine whether question wording and other techniques have to be changed to improve accurate disclosure among other social groups of lesbians. Efforts to measure reporting error should include standard quantitative and qualitative techniques, as well as techniques developed especially for this purpose. The use of ethnographic techniques to ascertain limits to validity may be especially useful.

Research should be funded and conducted to determine the best ways to ask questions about lesbian orientation, including the use of alternative wording and innovative technologies so as to obtain maximum disclosure. Such research should assess and measure the extent to which wordings appropriate for certain social groupings (e.g., women of specific racial or ethnic groups, social class, or regional groups) may be less appropriate for other groupings. This will allow investigators to minimize underreporting of lesbian status and also minimize biased estimates of the proportion of lesbians in different social groups.

Recommendation 3: Researchers should routinely consider including questions about sexual orientation on data collection forms in relevant studies in the behavioral and biomedical sciences to capture the full range of female experience and to increase knowledge about associations between sexual orientation and health status.

Current methodologies allow collection of information on sexual orientation with sufficient precision to discover important relationships. Further, such questions have been used successfully in a number of research areas with different populations. For example, a question on sexual identity was included in the Nurses' Health Study II, a large national cohort study, without apparent loss of participation. Identity was the focus in this study because it was believed that sexual identity and social relationships, rather than sexual behavior, were more likely to be determinants of breast cancer and other core concerns of the study.

The committee recommends that consideration be given to including questions about sexual identity, behavior, and attraction or desire in ongoing and future federal studies. These would include, for example, studies in which an association between sexual orientation and health can be hypothesized or in which discrimination based on sexual orientation may result in differential access to health care services. As appropriate, multiple dimensions of sexual orientation should be assessed whenever possible. Further, the rationale for including each question should be addressed in the study. These studies include, but are by no means limited to, the National Health and Nutrition Examination Survey, the National Household Survey on Drug Abuse, the National Survey of Family Growth, the American Community Survey, and the Youth Risk Behavior Survey. Pilot studies are recommended to test the feasibility of including these questions, with careful attention given to protecting confidentiality and assessing response bias and its impact on disclosure.

The committee recommends that researchers submitting proposals for federally funded research, whether unsolicited R01s, responses to Program Announcements, or responses to Requests for Proposals, routinely evaluate whether they should include sexual orientation questions in their protocols, just as they would other sociodemographic variables. The National Institutes of Health (NIH) review groups should be encouraged to consider whether or not sexual orientation should be assessed in proposed studies, and recommend inclusion of this data field when it would strengthen the value of the results.

Recommendation 4: Researchers studying lesbian health should consider the full range of racial, ethnic, and soc-

ioeconomic diversity found among lesbians when designing studies on lesbian health; strive to include members of the lesbian study population under study in the development and conduct of research; and give special attention to protecting the confidentiality and privacy of the study population.

There are a number of important considerations for conducting research on lesbian health. Because there are wide social and cultural differences in the health-related stressors, risks, and protective factors to which lesbians are exposed in different social and cultural milieus, the committee recommends that studies of lesbian health be funded that include the full range of variation in race and ethnicity, social class, age, and socioeconomic status.

Particularly given the lack of knowledge about lesbian health issues, the committee believes that it is imperative that researchers strive to involve members of the lesbian population being studied in the development and conduct of research on lesbian health. This is particularly important for identifying lesbians to include in research samples and for securing their participation. Involvement of the target population may take many forms and may occur at various stages of the research process, including the interpretation of research results. The committee further urges researchers to disseminate the results of their research studies to research participants.

The committee also recommends that special attention be given to ensure both confidentiality and the protection of human subjects in lesbian health research. This could be accomplished through a variety of mechanisms, including highlighting the unique ethical and research considerations in lesbian research to researchers and members of institutional review boards.

Recommendation 5: A large-scale probability survey should be funded to determine the range of expression of sexual orientation among all women and the prevalence of various risk and protective factors for health, by sexual orientation.

To date no large-scale probability studies on health have been conducted that collect information on sexual orientation. Conducting such a study would greatly increase knowledge about and understanding of sexual orientation in women, and improve understanding of the relationships among the dimensions of sexual orientation and health status and health behaviors.

Recommendation 6: Conferences should be held on an ongoing basis to disseminate information about the conduct and results of research on lesbian health, including the protection of human subjects.

The committee recommends that NIH and the Centers for Disease Control and Prevention (CDC) support periodic multidisciplinary conferences on lesbian health research methods and results. The first of these conferences should take place within the next two years, with subsequent meetings to take place on a regular basis. A model for such a conference is provided by the Conferences on Health Survey Methods at which researchers are convened to discuss the state of the art in a particular area of survey methodology. These conferences, which are convened periodically when the need arises for discussion of particular issues, have the objective of improving the quality of health survey data and enhancing their value and use by policy makers responsible for shaping health practice, policy, and programs (National Center for Health Statistics, 1996).

Given that the field of lesbian health research is still in its infancy and many researchers and members of institutional review boards are not aware of the ethical issues that should be considered in the conduct of research on lesbian health, the committee further urges that the NIH, in collaboration with the CDC, sponsor a conference on the ethical issues involved in conducting research on lesbian health, including issues related to privacy and confidentiality, future use of data, recruitment of subjects, and informed consent. This conference would be designed to inform members of institutional review boards, researchers, and members of federal review panels and should involve representatives from the lesbian community. One suggested mechanism for disseminating this information is through the National Human Subjects Protections Education Workshop Program conducted by the NIH Office of Protection from Research Risks. The committee encourages that the ethical issues involved in conducting research with lesbians be included as a topic for these workshops, which are held periodically at universities across the country.

Recommendation 7: Federal agencies, including the National Institutes of Health and the Centers for Disease Control and Prevention, foundations, health professional associations, and academic institutions, should develop and support mechanisms for broadly disseminating information about lesbian health to health care providers, researchers, and the public.

The committee recommends that mechanisms be developed to disseminate knowledge and state-of-the-art methodological strategies for designing and implementing lesbian health studies to researchers and students in academic and nonacademic research institutions and community settings.

The committee recommends the funding of a clearinghouse for research on lesbian health to make both published and unpublished research (e.g., conference papers) available to researchers and the public, including lesbian organizations. The committee further recommends that the clearinghouse make this information available via the World Wide Web as well as other means. The committee also recommends that health and mental health professional organizations feature discussions of lesbian health and the conduct of lesbian health research at their annual meetings. The committee notes that many of these organizations already have committees, caucuses, or divisions that focus on lesbian, gay, or bisexual issues.

Training programs on lesbian health and the special issues involved in working with lesbians should be implemented across a wide range of providers, including pediatricians, psychologists, substance abuse counselors and other treatment staff, general practitioners, obstetricians and gynecologists, psychiatrists, and social workers. The committee recommends that curricula be developed and implemented to train health care providers in offering guidance regarding sexuality, including homosexuality, to adolescents and their families.

Recommendation 8: The committee encourages development of strategies to train researchers in conducting lesbian health research at both the predoctoral and the postdoctoral levels.

Surveys of lesbians in academic settings and of graduate students indicate that individuals interested in conducting research on issues affecting lesbians face numerous barriers. In addition to the personal stigma sometimes experienced, it is difficult to find mentors or sponsors for research and to secure the funding support needed. The availability of training funds would increase the ability of young researchers to pursue careers in lesbian health research and would enhance their skills in managing the challenges of conducting this research.

A variety of strategies might be used to increase training opportunities for lesbian health researchers—for example, including lesbian health in the scope of pre- and postdoctoral programs in all health professions. NIH institutes could consider targeting training grants on lesbian health or including lesbian research in the scope of existing training grants. Further, foundations and academic institutions should consider providing training support in this area.

REFERENCE

National Center for Health Statistics. 1996. *Health Survey Research Methods: Conference Proceedings.* DHHS Pub. No. (PHS) 96-1013. Hyattsville, MD: U.S. Department of Health and Human Services.

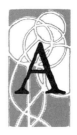

Selected Bibliography on Lesbian Health Research

This bibliography represents a compilation of research and other publications related to lesbian health. It includes references identified using the Medline and PsycLIT databases, as well as non-published material submitted to the committee. Although the bibliography is comprehensive, it is not exhaustive. Nonetheless, the committee believes that it is the most comprehensive and up-to-date bibliography currently available on lesbian health.

As an aid to the reader, references are organized into general categories. Thus, readers wishing to identify articles that cut across topics should check for them under multiple headings. Articles that do not fit into one of the specific topics (either because they cover many areas, or because they cover a unique or specific topic) are grouped together in the "general" category.

GENERAL

Bailey JM, Pillard RC, Kitzinger C, Wilkinson S. 1997. Sexual orientation: Is it determined by biology? In: Walsh MR, ed. *Women, Men, and Gender: Ongoing Debates*. New Haven, CT: Yale University Press. Pp. 181–203.
Blumstein P, Swartz P. 1983. *American Couples: Money, Work, Sex*. New York: William Morrow.

Bogaert AF. 1997. Birth order and sexual orientation in women. *Behavioral Neuroscience* 111(6):1395–1397.

Buunk BP, van Driel B. 1989. *Variant Lifestyles and Relationships*. Newbury Park, CA: Sage Publications.

Case P, Spiegelman D, Hunter DJ, Manson JE, Willet WC. 1996. *Sexual Orientation in Relation to Behaviors in the Nurses' Health Study II: Selected Results from a Pilot Study*. Presentation to the American Public Health Association. New York: National Development & Research Institutes.

Connolly L. 1996. Long-term care and hospice: The special needs of older gay men and lesbians. In: Peterson KJ, ed. *Health Care for Lesbians and Gay Men: Confronting Homophobia and Heterosexism*. New York: Harrington Park Press/Haworth Press. Pp. 79–91.

Cotton P. 1993. Gay, lesbian physicians meet, march, tell Shalala bigotry is health hazard [news]. *Journal of the American Medical Association* 269(20):2611–2612.

D'Augelli AR, Patterson CJ, eds. 1995. *Lesbian, Gay, and Bisexual Identities over the Lifespan: Psychological Perspectives*. New York: Oxford University Press.

Esterberg KG. 1990. From illness to action: Conceptions of homosexuality in *The Ladder*, 1956–1965. Special Issue: Feminist perspectives on sexuality. *Journal of Sex Research* 27(1):65–80.

Faderman L. 1978. The morbidification of love between women by 19th-century sexologists. *Journal of Homosexuality* 4(1):73–90.

Franklin S. 1993. Essentialism, which essentialism? Some implications of reproductive and genetic techno-science. *Journal of Homosexuality* 24(3–4):27–39.

Garnets LD, D'Augelli AR. 1994. Empowering lesbian and gay communities: A call for collaboration with community psychology. *American Journal of Community Psychology* 22(4):447–470.

Greene B. 1994. Lesbian and gay sexual orientations. In: Greene B, Herek GM, eds. *Lesbian and Gay Psychology: Theory, Research, and Clinical Applications*, Vol. 1. Thousand Oaks, CA: Sage Publications. Pp. 1–24.

Griffin G, ed. 1995. *Feminist Activism in the 1990s*. London: Taylor and Francis.

Haas AP, Hughes TL, Emanuel E, McCauley M. 1997. Building a lesbian health database. *National Lesbian and Gay Health Association: Conference Proceedings*. Washington, DC: National Lesbian and Gay Health Association.

Hale J. 1996. Blurring boundaries, making boundaries: Who is lesbian? *Journal of Homosexuality* 32(1):21–42.

Hall JA, Kimura D. 1995. Sexual orientation and performance on sexually dimorphic motor tasks. *Archives of Sexual Behavior* 24(4):395–407.

Herdt G, Boxer A. 1995. Bisexuality: Toward a comparative theory of identities and culture. In: Parker RG, Gagnon JH, eds. *Conceiving Sexuality: Approaches to Sex Research in a Postmodern World*. New York: Routledge. Pp. 63–89.

Hester SR, Biddle BS. 1995. Lesbian health invisible to mainstream [interview]. *AWHONN Voice* 3(2):10, 13.

Hollander J, Haber L. 1992. Ecological transition: Using Bronfenbrenner's model to study sexual identity change. Special Issue: Lesbian health: What are the issues? *Health Care for Women International* 13(2):121–129.

Hollander J, Haber L. 1993. Ecological transition: Using Bronfenbrenner's model to study sexual identity change. In: Stern, P ed. *Lesbian Health: What Are the Issues?* Washington, DC: Taylor and Francis. Pp. 31–39.

Hu S, Pattatucci AM, Patterson C, Li L, Fulker DW, Cherny SS, Kruglyak L, Hamer DH. 1995. Linkage between sexual orientation and chromosome Xq28 in males but not in females. *Nature Genetics* 11(3):248–256.

Jones WK. 1997. Personal communication. Washington, DC: Centers for Disease Control and Prevention, September 19.

Jordon JV, Kaplan AG, Miller JB, Stiver IP, Surrey JL. 1991. *Women's Growth in Connection.* New York: Guilford Press.

Kato PM, Mann T, eds. 1996. *Handbook of Diversity Issues in Health Psychology.* New York: Plenum Press.

Kenyon FE. 1968. Studies in female homosexuality, VI: The exclusively homosexual group. *Acta Psychiatrica Scandinavica* 44(3):224–237.

Kripke CC, Vaias L, Elliott A. 1994. The importance of taking a sensitive sexual history. *Journal of the American Medical Association* 271(9):713.

LaRosa JH. 1986. Executive women and health: Perceptions and practices. *American Journal of Public Health* 80:1450–1454.

Laumann EO, Michael RT, Gagnon JH. 1994. A political history of the national sex survey of adults. *Family Planning Perspectives* 26(1):34–38.

Lesbian Health Advocacy Network. 1995. *Recommendations of the Lesbian Health Advocacy Network.* Presented to the U.S. Public Health Service Women's Health Coordinators Meeting. Washington, DC: Lesbian Health Advocacy Network.

LeVay S, Nonas E. 1995. *City of Friends: A Portrait of the Gay and Lesbian Community in America.* Cambridge, MA: MIT Press.

Maggiore DJ. 1992. *Lesbianism: An Annotated Bibliography and Guide to the Literature, 1976–1991.* Metuchen, NJ: Scarecrow Press.

Matrix S. 1996. Desire and deviate nymphos: Performing inversion(s) as a lesbian consumer. *Journal of Homosexuality* 31(1–2):71–81.

McConnell JH. 1994. Lesbian and gay male identities as paradigms. In: Archer SL, ed. *Interventions for Adolescent Identity Development,* Vol. 169. Thousand Oaks, CA: Sage Publications. Pp. 103–118.

McCormick CM, Witelson SF. 1994. Functional cerebral asymmetry and sexual orientation in men and women. *Behavioral Neuroscience* 108(3):525–531.

McFadden D, Pasanen EG. 1998. Comparison of the auditory systems of heterosexuals and homosexuals: Click-evoked otoacoustic emissions. *Proceedings of the National Academy of Sciences of the USA* 95(5):2709–2713.

Money J. 1985. Pediatric sexology and hermaphroditism. *Journal of Sex and Marital Therapy* 11(3):139–156.

Money J. 1993. *The Adam Principle: Genes, Genitals, Hormones, and Gender: Selected Readings in Sexology.* Buffalo, NY: Prometheus Books.

Morrow DF. 1996. Coming-out issues for adult lesbians: A group intervention. *Social Work* 41(6):647–656.

National Gay and Lesbian Task Force. 1993. *Lesbian Health Issues and Recommendations.* Washington, DC: National Gay and Lesbian Task Force.

National Gay and Lesbian Task Force. 1998. Capital Gains and Losses '97: A State by State Review of All Gay, Lesbian, Bisexual and Transgender Legislation in 1997. Review by Issue [WWW Document]. URL http://www.ngltf.org/97cgal/review.html (accessed February 12, 1998).

National Research Council. 1997. *Evaluating Genetic Diversity*. Washington, DC: National Academy Press.

Pattatucci AM, Hamer DH. 1995. Development and familiality of sexual orientation in females. *Behavior Genetics* 25(5):407–420.

Patterson CJ. 1998. Sexual orientation and fertility. *Infertility in the Modern World. A Conference of the Cambridge Biosocial Society,* Cambridge, England, May 8.

Paul JP. 1996. Bisexuality: Exploring/exploding the boundaries. In: Savin-Williams RC, Cohen KM, eds. *The Lives of Lesbians, Gays, and Bisexuals: Children to Adults*. Fort Worth, TX: Harcourt Brace College Publishers. Pp. 436–461.

Pennaloza L. 1996. We're here, we're queer, and we're going shopping! A critical perspective on the accommodation of gays and lesbians in the U.S. marketplace. *Journal of Homosexuality* 31(1–2):9–41.

Peters DK, Cantrell PJ. 1991. Factors distinguishing samples of lesbians and heterosexual women. *Journal of Homosexuality* 21:1–15.

Peters DK, Cantrell PJ. 1993. Gender roles and role conflict in feminist lesbian and heterosexual women. *Sex Roles* 28(7/8):379–392.

Pierce RA, Black MA, eds. 1993. *Life-Span Development: A Diversity Reader*. Dubuque, IA: Kendall/Hunt Publishing Co.

Pilkington NW, Cantor JM. 1996. Perceptions of heterosexual bias in professional psychology programs: A survey of graduate students. *Professional Psychology: Research and Practice* 27(6):604–612.

Pisarski A, Gallois C. 1996. A needs analysis of Brisbane lesbians: Implications for the lesbian community. *Journal of Homosexuality* 30(4):79–95.

Platzer H. 1993. Ethics: Nursing care of gay and lesbian patients. *Nursing Standard* 7(17):34–37.

Plumb M. 1997. Statement of the Gay and Lesbian Medical Association to the IOM Committee on Lesbian Health Research Priorities Regarding Community Perspective, Washington, DC, July 23.

Pope M. 1995. The "salad bowl" is big enough for us all: An argument for the inclusion of lesbians and gay men in any definition of multiculturalism. *Journal of Counseling and Development* 73(3):301–304.

Purcell DW, Hicks DW. 1996. Institutional discrimination against lesbians, gay men, and bisexuals: The courts, legislature, and the military. Classics in lesbian studies. In: Cabaj RP, Stein TS, eds. *Textbook of Homosexuality and Mental Health*. Washington, DC: American Psychiatric Press. Pp. 763–782.

Rankow EJ. 1995. *Lesbian Health Bibliography*. San Francisco, CA: National Center for Lesbian Rights.

Rankow EJ. 1997. Primary medical care of the gay or lesbian patient. *North Carolina Medical Journal* 58(2):92–96.

Robohm JS, Buttenheim M. 1996. The gynecological care experience of adult survivors of childhood sexual abuse: A preliminary investigation. *Women and Health* 24(3):59–75.

Robson R. 1994. Resisting the family: Repositioning lesbians in legal theory. Special Issue: Feminism and the law. *Signs* 19(4):975–996.

Rose P. 1993. Out in the open? Lesbianism. *Nursing Times* 89(30):50–52.

Rothblum ED. 1988. Introduction: Lesbianism as a model of a positive lifestyle for women. Special Issue: Lesbianism: Affirming nontraditional roles. *Women and Therapy* 8(1–2):1–12.

Rust PC. 1993. "Coming out" in the age of social constructionism: Sexual identity formation among lesbian and bisexual women. *Gender and Society* 7(1):50–77.

Ryan C, Bradford J. 1997. *Lesbian Research Network: Final Report—Year 1.* Richmond, VA: An Uncommon Legacy Foundation.

Saddul RB, Jr. 1996. Coming out: An overlooked concept. *Clinical Nurse Specialist* 10(1):2–5, 56.

Saghir MT, Robins E. 1973. *Male and Female Homosexuality: A Comprehensive Investigation.* Baltimore, MD: Williams and Wilkins.

Sankar A. 1985. Sisters and brothers, lovers and enemies: Marriage resistance in southern Kwangtung. Special Issue: Anthropology and homosexual behavior. *Journal of Homosexuality* 11(3–4):69–81.

Savin-Williams RC, Cohen KM. 1996. *The Lives of Lesbians, Gays, and Bisexuals: Children to Adults.* Fort Worth, TX: Harcourt Brace College Publishers.

Seeman TE, McEwen B. 1996. Impact of social environment characteristics on neuroendocrine regulation. *Psychosomatic Medicine* 58:459–471.

Shively MG, De Cecco JP. 1993. Components of sexual identity. In: Garnets LD, Kimmel DC, eds. *Psychological Perspectives on Lesbian and Gay Male Experience.* New York: Columbia University Press. Pp. 80–88.

Shore ER. 1990. Business and professional women: Primary prevention for new role incumbents. In: Roman PM, ed. *Alcohol Problem Intervention in the Workplace: Employee Assistance Programs and Strategic Alternatives.* New York: Quorum Press. Pp. 113–124.

Simpson LA. 1997. History of gay and lesbian physician groups. *Journal of the Gay and Lesbian Medical Association* 1(1):61–63.

Stephany TM. 1993. Lesbian hospice patients. *Home Healthcare Nurse* 11(6):65.

Stevens PE. 1994. Protective strategies of lesbian clients in health care environments. *Research in Nursing and Health* 17(3):217–229.

Stevens PE, Hall JM. 1991. A critical historical analysis of the medical construction of lesbianism. *International Journal of Health Services* 21(2):291–307.

Time. 1991. No sex, we're Republicans. *Time* August 5:27.

Troiden RR. 1988. Homosexual identity development. *Journal of Adolescent Health Care* 9:105–113.

Troiden RR. 1989. The formation of homosexual identities. *Journal of Homosexuality* 17:43–73.

Vacc NA, DeVaney SB, Wittmer J, eds. 1995. *Experiencing and Counseling Multicultural and Diverse Populations.* 3rd Edition. Muncie, IN: Accelerated Development.

Wegesin DJ. 1998. A neuropsychologic profile of homosexual and heterosexual men and women. *Archives of Sexual Behavior* 27(1):91–108.

Wolfe A. 1998. *One Nation, After All: What Americans Really Think About God, Country, Family, Racism, Welfare, Immigration, Homosexuality, Work, the Right, the Left and Each Other.* New York: Viking Press.

World Health Organization. 1946. *Constitution of the World Health Organization.* New York: International Health Conference.

World Health Organization. 1998. Definition of Health [WWW Document]. URL http://www.who.ch/aboutwho/definition.htm (accessed March 11, 1998).

ADOLESCENTS

Abinati A. 1994. Legal challenges facing lesbian and gay youth. In: DeCrescenzo T, ed. *Helping Gay and Lesbian Youth: New Policies, New Programs, New Practice.* New York: Harrington Park Press/Haworth Press, Inc. Pp. 149–169.

Bidwell RJ, Deisher RW. 1991. Adolescent sexuality: Current issues. *Pediatric Annals* 20(6):293–302.

Boxer AM, Cook JA, Herdt G. 1991. Double jeopardy: Identity transitions and parent–child relations among gay and lesbian youth. In: Pillemer KA, McCartney K, eds. *Parent–Child Relations Throughout Life.* Hillsdale, NJ: Lawrence Erlbaum Associates, Inc. Pp. 52–92.

Boxer AM, Cohler BJ, Herdt G, Irvin F. 1993. Gay and lesbian youth. In: Tolan PH, Cohler BJ, eds. *Handbook of Clinical Research and Practice with Adolescents.* New York: John Wiley and Sons. Pp. 249–280.

Braverman PK, Strasburger VC. 1993. Adolescent sexual activity. *Clinical Pediatrics* 32 (11):658–668.

Bridget J, Lucille S. 1996. Lesbian youth support information service (LYSIS): Developing a distance support agency for young lesbians. *Journal of Community and Applied Social Psychology* 6(5):355–364.

Buhrke RA, Stabb SD. 1995. Gay, lesbian, and bisexual student needs. In: Stabb SD, Harris SM, Talley JE, eds. *Multicultural Needs Assessment for College and University Student Populations.* Springfield, IL: Charles C. Thomas. Pp. 173–201.

Coleman E, Remafedi G. 1989. Gay, lesbian, and bisexual adolescents: A critical challenge to counselors. Special Issue: Gay, lesbian, and bisexual issues in counseling. *Journal of Counseling and Development* 68(1):36–40.

Creatsas GK. 1993. Sexuality: Sexual activity and contraception during adolescence. *Current Opinion in Obstetrics and Gynecology* 5(6):774–783.

D'Augelli AR. 1996. Lesbian, gay, and bisexual development during adolescence and young adulthood. In: Cabaj RP, Stein TS, eds. *Textbook of Homosexuality and Mental Health.* Washington, DC: American Psychiatric Press. Pp. 267–288.

D'Augelli AR, Ehrenberg M. 1996. Enhancing the development of lesbian, gay, and bisexual youths. Aging and mental health: Issues in the gay and lesbian community. In: Rothblum ED, Bond LA, eds. *Preventing Heterosexism and Homophobia. Primary Prevention of Psychopathology,* Vol. 17. New York: Harrington Park Press/Haworth Press. Pp. 189–209.

D'Augelli AR, Hershberger SL. 1993. Lesbian, gay, and bisexual youth in community settings: Personal challenges and mental health problems. *American Journal of Community Psychology* 21(4):421–448.

DeCrescenzo T, ed. 1994. *Helping Gay and Lesbian Youth: New Policies, New Programs, New Practice*. New York: Harrington Park Press/Haworth Press.

Dempsey CL. 1994. Health and social issues of gay, lesbian, and bisexual adolescents. *Families in Society* 75(3):160–167.

Durby DD. 1994. Gay, lesbian, and bisexual youth. In: DeCrescenzo T, ed. *Helping Gay and Lesbian Youth: New Policies, New Programs, New Practice*. New York: Harrington Park Press/Hayworth Press. Pp. 1–37.

Evans NJ, D'Augelli AR. 1996. Lesbians, gay men, and bisexual people in college. In: Savin-Williams RC, Cohen KM, eds. *The Lives of Lesbians, Gays, and Bisexuals: Children to Adults*. Fort Worth, TX: Harcourt Brace College Publishers. Pp. 201–226.

Feldman DA. 1989. Gay youth and AIDS. Special Issue: Gay and lesbian youth: I. *Journal of Homosexuality* 17(1–2):185–193.

Fine M. 1993. Sexuality, schooling, and adolescent females: The missing discourse of desire. In: Weis L, Fine M, eds. *Beyond Silenced Voices: Class, Race, and Gender in United States Schools*. Albany, NY: State University of New York Press. Pp. 75–99.

Fontaine JH, Hammond NL. 1996. Counseling issues with gay and lesbian adolescents. *Adolescence* 31(124):817–830.

French S, Story M, Remafedi G, Resnick M, Blum R. 1996. Sexual orientation and prevalence of body dissatisfaction and eating disordered behaviors: A population-based study of adolescents. *International Journal of Eating Disorders* 19(2):119–126.

Garofalo R, Wolf RC, Kessel S, Palfrey SJ, DuRant RH. 1998. The association between health risk behaviors and sexual orientation among a school-based sample of adolescents. *Pediatrics* 101(5):895–902.

Gochros HL, Bidwell R. 1996. Lesbian and gay youth in a straight world: Implications for health care workers. In: Peterson KJ, ed. *Health Care for Lesbians and Gay Men: Confronting Homophobia and Heterosexism*. New York: Harrington Park Press/Haworth Press. Pp. 1–17.

Gonsiorek JC. 1988. Mental health issues of gay and lesbian adolescents. *Journal of Adolescent Health Care* 9(2):114–122.

Gonsiorek JC. 1993. Mental health issues of gay and lesbian adolescents. In: Garnets LD, Kimmel DC, eds. *Psychological Perspectives on Lesbian and Gay Male Experiences. Between Men—Between Women: Lesbian and Gay Studies*. New York: Columbia University Press. Pp. 469–485.

Graber JA, Brooks-Gunn J. 1995. Models of development: Understanding risk in adolescence. *Suicide and Life-Threatening Behavior* 25(Suppl):18–25.

Grossman AH. 1994. Homophobia: A cofactor of HIV disease in gay and lesbian youth. *Journal of the Association of Nurses in AIDS Care* 5(1):39–43.

Gullotta TP, Adams GR, Montemayor R, eds. 1993. *Adolescent Sexuality*. Newbury Park, CA: Sage Publications.

Hunter J. 1990. Violence against lesbian and gay male youths. Special Issue: Violence against lesbians and gay men: Issues for research, practice, and policy. *Journal of Interpersonal Violence* 5(3):295–300.

Hunter J. 1995. At the crossroads: Lesbian youth. In: Jay K, ed. *From Growing Up to Growing Old—Dyke Life: A Celebration of the Lesbian Experience.* New York: Basics Books. Pp. 50–60.

Hunter J, Schaecher R. 1995. Gay and lesbian adolescents. In: Edwards RL, ed. *Encyclopedia of Social Work,* 19th Edition. Washington, DC: National Association of Social Workers. Pp. 1055–1063.

Kleis BN, Lock J. 1995. The public discussion of homosexuality. *Journal of the American Academy of Child and Adolescent Psychiatry* 34(1):6.

Kokotailo PK, Stephenson JN. 1993. Sexuality and reproductive health behavior. In: Singer MI, Singer LT, Anglin TM, eds. *Handbook for Screening Adolescents at Psychosocial Risk.* New York: Lexington Books/Macmillan. Pp. 249–292.

Kreiss JL, Patterson DL. 1997. Psychosocial issues in primary care of lesbian, gay, bisexual, and transgender youth. *Journal of Pediatric Health Care* 11(6):266–274.

Mallon G. 1992. Gay and no place to go: Assessing the needs of gay and lesbian adolescents in out-of-home care settings. *Child Welfare* 71(6):547–556.

Martin AD, Hetrick ES. 1988. The stigmatization of the gay and lesbian adolescent. *Journal of Homosexuality* 15(1–2):163–183.

Morrow DF. 1993. Social work with gay and lesbian adolescents [published erratum appears in *Social Work* 1994 39(2):166]. *Social Work* 38(6):655–660.

Nelson JA. 1997. Gay, lesbian, and bisexual adolescents: Providing esteem-enhancing care to a battered population. *Nursing Practice* 22(2):94, 99, 103 passim.

Owen WF. 1985. Medical problems of the homosexual adolescent. *Journal of Adolescent Health Care* 6(4):278–285.

Paroski PA, Jr. 1987. Health care delivery and the concerns of gay and lesbian adolescents. *Journal of Adolescent Health Care* 8(2):188–192.

Perrin E. 1996. Pediatricians and gay and lesbian youth [see comments]. *Pediatrics in Review* 17(9):311–318.

Petersen AC, Leffert N, Graham BL. 1995. Adolescent development and the emergence of sexuality. *Suicide and Life-Threatening Behavior* 25(Suppl):4–17.

Remafedi G. 1990. Fundamental issues in the care of homosexual youth. *Medical Clinics of North America* 74(5):1169–1179.

Saltzburg S. 1996. Family therapy and the disclosure of adolescent homosexuality. *Journal of Family Psychotherapy* 7(4):1–18.

Sanford ND. 1989. Providing sensitive health care to gay and lesbian youth. *Nurse Practitioner* 14(5):30–32, 35–36, 39 passim.

Savin-Williams RC. 1989. Gay and lesbian adolescents. *Marriage and Family Review* 14(3–4):197–216.

Savin-Williams RC. 1994. Verbal and physical abuse as stressors in the lives of lesbian, gay male, and bisexual youths: Associations with school problems, running away, substance abuse, prostitution, and suicide. Special Section: Mental health of lesbians and gay men. *Journal of Consulting and Clinical Psychology* 62(2):261–269.

Savin-Williams RC. 1996. Self-labeling and disclosure among gay, lesbian, and bisexual youths. In: Laird J, Green RJ, eds. *Lesbians and Gays in Couples and Families: A Handbook for Therapists.* San Francisco, CA: Jossey-Bass. Pp. 153–182.

Savin-Williams RC, Lenhart RE. 1990. AIDS prevention among gay and lesbian youth: Psychosocial stress and health care intervention guidelines. In: Ostrow DG, ed. *Behavioral Aspects of AIDS.* New York: Plenum Press. Pp. 75–99.

Savin-Williams RC, Rodriguez RG. 1993. A developmental, clinical perspective on lesbian, gay male, and bisexual youths. In: Gullotta TP, Adams GR, Montemayor R, eds. *Adolescent Sexuality. Advances in Adolescent Development.* Newbury Park, CA: Sage Publications. Pp. 77–101.

Schneider M. 1991. Developing services for lesbian and gay adolescents. *Canadian Journal of Community Mental Health* 10(1):133–151.

Schuster MA, Bell RM, Petersen LP, Kanouse DE. 1996. Communication between adolescents and physicians about sexual behavior and risk prevention. *Archives of Pediatrics and Adolescent Medicine* 150(9):906–913.

Sullivan TR. 1994. Obstacles to effective child welfare service with gay and lesbian youths. *Child Welfare* 73(4):291–304.

Teague JB. 1992. Issues relating to the treatment of adolescent lesbians and homosexuals. *Journal of Mental Health Counseling* 14(4):422–439.

Townsend MH, Wallick MM, Pleak RR, Cambre KM. 1997. Gay and lesbian issues in child and adolescent psychiatry training as reported by training directors. *Journal of the American Academy of Child and Adolescent Psychiatry* 36(6):764–768.

Travers R, Schneider M. 1996. Barriers to accessibility for lesbian and gay youth needing addictions services. *Youth & Society* 27(3):356–378.

Uribe V, Harbeck KM. 1992. Addressing the needs of lesbian, gay, and bisexual youth: The origins of PROJECT 10 and school-based intervention. *Journal of Homosexuality* 22(3–4):9–28.

AGING

Deevey S. 1990. Older lesbian women. An invisible minority. *Journal of Gerontological Nursing* 16(5):35–39.

Ehrenberg M. 1996. Aging and mental health: Issues in the gay and lesbian community. In: Alexander CJ, ed. *Gay and Lesbian Mental Health: A Sourcebook for Practitioners.* New York: Harrington Park Press/Haworth Press. Pp. 189–209.

Fullmer EM. 1995. Challenging biases against families of older gays and lesbians. In: Smith GC, Tobin SS, Robertson-Tchabo EA, Power PW, eds. *Strengthening Aging Families: Diversity in Practice and Policy.* Thousand Oaks, CA: Sage Publications. Pp. 99–119.

Kehoe M. 1986. Lesbians over 65: A triply invisible minority. *Journal of Homosexuality* 12(3–4):139–152.

Kehoe M. 1988. Lesbians over 60 speak for themselves. *Journal of Homosexuality* 16(3–4):1–111.

McDougall GJ. 1993. Therapeutic issues with gay and lesbian elders. Special Issue: The forgotten aged: Ethnic, psychiatric, and societal minorities. *Clinical Gerontologist* 14(1):45–57.

Rothblum ED, Ehrenberg M, Ehrenberg M. 1997. Classics in lesbian studies. Aging and mental health: Issues in the gay and lesbian community. In: Alexander CJ, ed. *Gay and Lesbian Mental Health: A Sourcebook for Practitioners.* New York: Harrington Park Press/Haworth Press. Pp. 189–209.

Slusher M, Mayer C, Dunkle R. 1996. Gays and Lesbians Older and Wiser (GLOW): A support group for older gay people. *Gerontologist* 36(1):118–123.

Turk Charles S, Rose T, Gatz M. 1996. The significance of gender in the treatment of older adults. In: Carstensen L, Edelstein B, Dornbrand L, eds. *The Practical Handbook of Clinical Gerontology*. Thousand Oaks, CA: Sage Publications.

Waite H, Ehrenberg M. 1995. Lesbians leaping out of the intergenerational contract: Issues of aging in Australia. Aging and mental health: Issues in the gay and lesbian community. In: Sullivan G, Leong LW-T, eds. *Gays and Lesbians in Asia and the Pacific: Social and Human Services*. New York: Harrington Park Press/Haworth Press. Pp. 109–127.

ATTITUDES AND HOMOPHOBIA

Berkman CS, Zinberg G. 1997. Homophobia and heterosexism in social workers. *Social Work* 42(4):319–332.

Brogan M. 1997. Healthcare for lesbians: Attitudes and experiences. *Nursing Standards* 11(45):39–42.

Davies D. 1996. Homophobia and heterosexism. In: Davise D, Neal C, eds. *Pink Therapy: A Guide for Counselors and Therapists Working with Lesbian, Gay and Bisexual Clients*. Buckingham, England: Open University Press. Pp. 41–65.

Druzin P, Shrier I, Yacowar M, Rossignol M. 1998. Discrimination against gay, lesbian and bisexual family physicians by patients. *Canadian Medical Association Journal* 158(5):593–597.

Eliason MJ. 1996. A survey of the campus climate for lesbian, gay, and bisexual university members. *Journal of Psychology and Human Sexuality* 8(4):39–58.

Eliason MJ, Donelan C, Randall C. 1992. Lesbian stereotypes. Special Issue: Lesbian health: What are the issues? *Health Care for Women International* 13(2):131–144.

Eliason MJ. 1997. The prevalence and nature of biphobia in heterosexual undergraduate students. *Archives of Sexual Behavior* 26(3):317–326.

Eliason MJ. 1998. Correlates of prejudice in nursing students. *Journal of Nursing Education* 37(1):27–29.

Eliason MJ, Randall CE. 1991. Lesbian phobia in nursing students. *Western Journal of Nursing Research* 13(3):363–374.

Faria G. 1997. The challenge of health care social work with gay men and lesbians. *Social Work in Health Care* 25(1–2):65–72.

Garfinkle E, Morin SF. 1978. Psychologists' attitudes toward homosexual psychotherapy clients. *Journal of Social Issues* 34(3):101–112.

Gray DP, Kramer M, Minick P, McGehee L, Thomas D, Greiner D. 1996. Heterosexism in nursing education. *Journal of Nursing Education* 35(5):204–210.

Israelstam S. 1988. Knowledge and opinions of alcohol intervention workers in Ontario, Canada, regarding issues affecting male gays and lesbians: Parts I and II. *International Journal of the Addictions* 23(3):227–252.

Long JK. 1996. Working with lesbians, gays, and bisexuals: Addressing heterosexism in supervision [see comments]. *Family Process* 35(3):377–388.

Mallet P, Apostolidis T, Paty B. 1997. The development of gender schemata about hetero-sexual and homosexual others during adolescence. *Journal of General Psychology* 124(1):91–104.

Mathews WC, Booth M, Turner JD, Kessler L. 1986. Physicians' attitudes toward homo-sexuality: Survey of a California County Medical Society. *Western Journal of Medicine* 144:106–110.

McDermott RJ, Drolet JC, Fetro JV. 1989. Connotative meanings of sexuality-related terms: Implications for educators and other practitioners. *Journal of Sex Education and Therapy* 15(2):103–113.

McHenry SS, Johnson JW. 1993. Homophobia in the therapist and gay or lesbian client: Conscious and unconscious collusions in self-hate. *Psychotherapy* 30(1):141–151.

McKee MB, Hayes SF, Axiotis IR. 1994. Challenging heterosexism in college health service delivery. *Journal of American College Health* 42(5):211–216.

McNaron TAH. 1997. *Poisoned Ivy: Lesbian and Gay Academics Confronting Homophobia.* Philadelphia: Temple University Press.

Messing AE, Schoenberg R, Stephens RK. 1983. Confronting homophobia in health care settings: Guidelines for social work practice. *Journal of Social Work and Human Sexuality* 2(2–3):65–74.

Morrissey M. 1996. Attitudes of practitioners to lesbian, gay and bisexual clients. *British Journal of Nursing* 5(16):980–982.

Nelson ES, Krieger SL. 1997. Changes in attitudes toward homosexuality in college stu-dents: Implementation of a gay men and lesbian peer panel. *Journal of Homosexuality* 33(2):63–81.

O'Hanlan KA. 1995. Lesbian health and homophobia: Perspectives for the treating obste-trician/gynecologist. *Current Problems in Obstetrics, Gynecology and Fertility* 18(4):93–136.

O'Hanlan KA. 1996. Homophobia and the health psychology of lesbians. In: Kato PM, Mann T, eds. *Handbook of Diversity Issues in Health Psychology.* New York: Plenum Press. Pp. 261–284.

O'Hanlan KA, Cabaj RP, Schatz B, Lock J, Nemrow P. 1997. A review of the medical consequences of homophobia with suggestions for resolution. *Journal of the Gay and Lesbian Medical Association* 1(1):25–39.

Oriel KA, Madlon-Kay DJ, Govaker D, Mersy DJ. 1996. Gay and lesbian physicians in training: Family practice program directors' attitudes and students' perceptions of bias. *Family Medicine* 28(10):720–725.

Peterson KJ, ed. 1996. *Health Care for Lesbians and Gay Men: Confronting Homophobia and Heterosexism.* New York: Harrington Park Press/Haworth Press.

Peterson KJ, Bricker JM. 1996. Lesbians and the health care system. In: Peterson KJ, ed. *Health Care for Lesbians and Gay Men: Confronting Homophobia and Heterosexism.* New York: Harrington Park Press/Hayworth Press. Pp. 33–47.

Polansky JS, Karasic DH, Speier PL, Hastik K, Haller E. 1997. Homophobia: Therapeutic and training considerations for psychiatry. *Journal of the Gay and Lesbian Medical Asso-ciation* 1(1):41–47.

Ramos MM, Tellez CM, Palley TB, Umland BE, Skipper BJ. 1998. Attitudes of physi-cians practicing in New Mexico toward gay men and lesbians in the profession. *Academic Medicine* 73(4):436–438.

Randall CE. 1989. Lesbian phobia among BSN educators: A survey. *Journal of Nursing Education* 28(7):302–306.

Robb N. 1996. Fear of ostracism still silences some gay MDs, students [see comments]. *Canadian Medical Association Journal* 155(7):972–977.

Rose P, Platzer H. 1993. Confronting prejudice. Gay and lesbian issues. *Nursing Times* 89(31):52–54.

Rothblum ED, Bond LA, eds. 1996. *Preventing Heterosexism and Homophobia*. Thousand Oaks, CA: Sage Publications.

Rudolph J. 1989. Effects of a workshop on mental health practitioners' attitudes toward homosexuality and counseling effectiveness. Special Issue: Gay, lesbian, and bisexual issues in counseling. *Journal of Counseling and Development* 68(1):81–85.

Schatz B, O'Hanlan KA. 1994. *Anti-Gay Discrimination in Medicine: Results of a National Survey of Lesbian, Gay and Bisexual Physicians*. San Francisco, CA: American Association of Physicians for Human Rights (AAPHR).

Schwanberg SL. 1985. Changes in labeling homosexuality in health sciences literature: A preliminary investigation. *Journal of Homosexuality* 12(1):51–73.

Schwanberg SL. 1990. Attitudes towards homosexuality in American health care literature 1983–1987. *Journal of Homosexuality* 19(3):117–136.

Schwanberg SL. 1996. Health care professionals' attitudes toward lesbian women and gay men. *Journal of Homosexuality* 31(3):71–83.

Sharkey L. 1987. Nurses in the closet: Is nursing open and receptive to gay and lesbian nurses? *Imprint* 34(3):38–39.

Simkin RJ. 1993. Creating openness and receptiveness with your patients: Overcoming heterosexual assumptions. *Canadian Journal of Ob/Gyn and Women's Health Care* 5(4):485–489.

Simon A. 1995. Some correlates of individuals' attitudes toward lesbians. *Journal of Homosexuality* 29(1):89–103.

Smith EM, Johnson SR, Guenther SM. 1985. Health care attitudes and experiences during gynecologic care among lesbians and bisexuals. *American Journal of Public Health* 75(9):1085–1087.

Smith GB. 1993. Homophobia and attitudes toward gay men and lesbians by psychiatric nurses. *Archives of Psychiatric Nursing* 7(6):377–384.

Stevens PE, Booth M, Turner J, Kessler D. 1994. Physicians' attitudes toward homosexuality—Survey of a California county medical society. *Western Journal of Nursing Research* 16(6):639–659.

Wagner L. 1997. Lesbian health and homophobia. *Tennessee Nurse* 60(4):15–16.

Waldo CR, Kemp JL. 1997. Should I come out to my students? An empirical investigation. *Journal of Homosexuality* 34(2):79–94.

Walpin L. 1997. Combating heterosexism: Implications for nursing. *Clinical Nurse Specialist* 11(3):126–132.

Wilkerson A. 1994. Homophobia and the moral authority of medicine. *Journal of Homosexuality* 27(3–4):329–347.

CANCER

Bicker-Jenkins M. 1994. Feminist practice and breast cancer: "The patriarchy has claimed my right breast. . . ." *Social Work in Health Care* 19(3–4):17–42.

Campbell K. 1996. CDC targets lesbians for cancer screening. *The Washington Blade* January 6, pp. 1, 21.

Capen K. 1997. Can doctors place limits on their medical practices? *Canadian Medical Association Journal* 156(6):839–840.

Community Liaison Program. 1994. *Cancer and Cancer Risk Among Lesbians: Proceedings of an Interactive Working Conference,* Seattle, WA, December 2–3. Seattle: Fred Hutchinson Cancer Research Center.

Denenberg R. 1994. I'm gay, so why do I need a Pap smear? *LAP Notes* Spring:8.

Ferris DG, Batish S, Wright TC, Cushing C, Scott EH. 1996. A neglected lesbian health concern: Cervical neoplasia. *Journal of Family Practice* 43(6):581–584.

Haber S, Acuff C, Ayers L, Freeman EL, Goodheart C, Kieffer CC, Lubin LB, Mikesell SG, Siegel M, et al. 1995. *Breast Cancer: A Psychological Treatment Manual.* New York: Springer.

Matthews AK. 1998. Lesbians and cancer support: Clinical issues for cancer patients. *Health Care for Women International* 19(3):193–203.

Mullineaux DG, French SA. 1997. Lesbian couples and cancer. *Nebraska Nurse* 30(3):30–31.

Ott C, Eilers J. 1997. Breast cancer and women partnering with women. *Nebraska Nurse* 30(3):29.

Price JH, Easton AN, Telljohann SK, Wallace PB. 1996. Perceptions of cervical cancer and Pap smear screening behavior by women's sexual orientation. *Journal of Community Health* 21(2):89–105.

Rankow EJ. 1995a. Breast and cervical cancer among lesbians. *Women's Health Issues* 5(3):123–129.

DRUG ABUSE

Barthwell AG. 1997. Cultural considerations in the management of addictive disease. In: Miller NS, Gold MS, Smith DE, eds. *Manual of Therapeutics for Addictions.* New York: Wiley-Liss. Pp. 246–254.

Bidwell RJ. 1986. Lesbian alcoholics. *Social Work* 31(3):238.

Bloomfield K. 1993. A comparison of alcohol consumption between lesbians and heterosexual women in an urban population. *Drug and Alcohol Dependence* 33:257–269.

Cabaj RP. 1992. Gays, lesbians, and bisexuals. In: Lowinson J, Ruiz P, Millman R, Langrod J, eds. *Substance Abuse: A Comprehensive Textbook.* 3rd Edition. Baltimore, MD: Williams and Wilkins. Pp. 725–733.

Cabaj RP. 1992. Substance abuse in the gay and lesbian community. In: Lowenson J, Ruiz P, Millman R, eds. *Substance Abuse: A Comprehensive Textbook.* Baltimore, MD: Williams and Wilkins. Pp. 852–860.

Cabaj RP. 1996. Substance abuse in gay men, lesbians, and bisexuals. In: Cabaj RP, Stein TS, eds. *Textbook of Homosexuality and Mental Health.* Washington, DC: American Psychiatric Press, Inc. Pp. 783–799.

Covington SS, Surey JL. 1997. The relational model of women's psychological development: Implications for substance abuse. In: Wilsnack RW, Wilsnack SC, eds. *Gender and Alcohol: Individual and Social Perspectives.* New Brunswick, NJ: Rutgers Center of Alcohol Studies. Pp. 335–351.

Fifield LH, Latham JD, Phillips C. 1977. Alcoholism in the Gay Community: The Price of Alienation, Isolation, and Oppression. Unpublished monograph. Los Angeles, CA: Gay Community Services Center.

Finnegan DG, McNally EB. 1990. Lesbian women. In: Engs RC, ed. *Women: Alcohol and Other Drugs.* Dubuque, IA: Kendall/Hunt Publishing Company. Pp. 149–156.

Glaus KO. 1989. Alcoholism, chemical dependency and the lesbian client. *Women and Therapy* 8(2):131–144.

Hall JM. 1990. Alcoholism in lesbians: Developmental, symbolic interactionist, and critical perspectives. *Health Care for Women International* 11(1):89–107.

Hall JM. 1990. Alcoholism recovery in lesbian women: A theory in development. *Scholarly Inquiry in Nursing Practice* 4(2):109–122; discussion 123–125.

Hall JM. 1992. An exploration of lesbians' images of recovery from alcohol problems. *Health Care for Women International* 13(2):181–198.

Hall JM. 1992. Lesbians' Experiences with Alcohol Problems: A Critical Ethnographic Study of Problematization, Helpseeking and Recovery Patterns. Dissertation abstract, University of California, San Francisco.

Hall JM. 1993. Lesbians and alcohol: Patterns and paradoxes in medical notions and lesbians' beliefs. *Journal of Psychoactive Drugs* 25(2):109–119.

Hall JM. 1993. What really worked? A case analysis and discussion of confrontational intervention for substance abuse in marginalized women. *Archives of Psychiatric Nursing* 7(6):322–327.

Hall JM. 1994. Lesbians recovering from alcohol problems: An ethnographic study of health care experiences. *Nursing Research* 43(4):238–244.

Hall JM. 1994. The experiences of lesbians in Alcoholics Anonymous. Special Issue: Feminist research methods in nursing research. *Western Journal of Nursing Research* 16(5):556–576.

Hall JM. 1996. Pervasive effects of childhood sexual abuse in lesbians' recovery from alcohol problems. *Substance Use and Misuse* 31(2):225–239.

Hellman RE, Staton M, Lee J, Tytun A, Vachon R. 1989. Treatment of homosexual alcoholics in government-funded agencies: Provider training and attitudes. *Hospital and Community Psychiatry* 40(11):1163–1168.

Hesselbrock MN, Hesselbrock VM. 1997. Gender, alcoholism, and psychiatric comorbidity. In: Wilsnack RW, Wilsnack SC, eds. *Gender and Alcohol: Individual and Social Perspectives.* New Brunswick, NJ: Rutgers Center of Alcohol Studies. Pp. 49–71.

Hughes TL, Flay B. In progress. Gender roles and substance abuse: A theoretical perspective.

Hughes TL, Norris J. 1995. Sexuality, sexual orientation and violence: Missing pieces in the puzzle of women's abuse of alcohol. In: McElmurry B, Parker R, eds. *Annual Review of Women's Health,* Vol. 2. New York: National League for Nursing. Pp. 285–317.

Hughes TL, Wilsnack SC. 1994. Research on lesbians and alcohol: Gaps and implications. *Alcohol Health and Research World* 18(3):202–205.

Hughes TL, Wilsnack SC. 1997. Use of alcohol among lesbians: Research and clinical implications. *American Journal of Orthopsychiatry* 67(1):20–36.

Hughes TL, Day LE, Marcantonio R, Torpy E. 1997. Gender differences in alcohol and other drug use in young adults. *Substance Use and Misuse* 32(3):319–344.

Israelstam S, Lambert S. 1986. Homosexuality and alcohol: Observation and research after the psychoanalytic era. *International Journal of the Addictions* 21(4–5):509–537.

McKirnan DJ, Peterson PL. 1989. Alcohol and drug use among homosexual men and women: Epidemiology and population characteristics. *Addictive Behaviors* 14:545–553.

McKirnan DJ, Peterson PL. 1989. Psychosocial and cultural factors in alcohol and drug abuse: An analysis of a homosexual population. *Addictive Behaviors* 14:555–563.

Nadeau L. 1990. Alcoholism, mental health and homosexuality: 3 female lesbian cases. *Sante Mentale au Quebec* 15(1):237–243.

Neisen JH, Sandall H. 1990. Alcohol and other drug abuse in gay/lesbian populations: Related to victimization? *Journal of Psychology and Human Sexuality* 3(1):151–168.

Nicoloff LK, Stiglitz E. 1987. Lesbian alcoholism: Etiology, treatment, and recovery. In: Boston Lesbian Psychologies Collective, eds. *Lesbian Psychologies.* Chicago: University of Illinois Press. Pp. 283–293.

Norris J, Hughes TL. 1996. Alcohol consumption and female sexuality: A review. In: Howard JM, Martin SE, Mail PD, Hilton ME, Taylor ED, eds. *Women and Alcohol: Issues for Prevention Research.* Research Monograph No. 32. Bethesda, MD: National Institutes of Health, National Institute on Alcohol Abuse and Alcoholism. Pp. 315–345.

Perry SM. 1995. Lesbian alcohol and marijuana use: Correlates of HIV risk behaviors and abusive relationships. *Journal of Psychoactive Drugs* 27(4):413–419.

Romans-Clarkson SE, Walton VA, Herbison GP, Mullen PE. 1992. Alcohol-related problems in New Zealand women. *Australian and New Zealand Journal of Psychiatry* 26:175–182.

Schilit R, Lie G, Montagne M. 1990. Substance abuse as a correlate of violence in intimate lesbian relationships. *Journal of Homosexuality* 19(3):51–65.

Shernoff M, Springer E. 1992. Substance abuse and AIDS: Report from the front lines (the impact on professionals). Special Issue: Lesbians and gay men: Chemical dependency treatment issues. *Journal of Chemical Dependency Treatment* 5(1):35–48.

Skinner WF. 1994. The prevalence and demographic predictors of illicit and licit drug use among lesbians and gay men. *American Journal of Public Health* 84(8):1307–1310.

Skinner WF, Otis MD. 1996. Drug and alcohol use among lesbian and gay people in a southern U.S. sample: Epidemiological, comparative, and methodological findings from the Triology Project. *Journal of Homosexuality* 30(3):59–92.

Solis-Marich and Associates. 1994. *Recommendations on Access to Substance Abuse Services for the Lesbian and Gay Communities.* Submitted to the Center for Substance Abuse Treatment (CSAT). Washington, DC: Lesbian and Gay Substance Abuse Workgroup.

Underhill BL. 1991. Recovery needs of lesbian alcoholics in treatment. In: Van Den Bergh N, ed. *Feminist Perspectives on Addictions*. New York: Springer Publishing Co. Pp. 73–86.

Weathers B. 1980. Alcoholism and the lesbian community. In: Eddy CC, Ford JL, eds. *Alcoholism in Women*. Dubuque, IA: Kendall/Hunt Publishing Company. Pp. 142–149.

Weinstein D, ed. 1992. *Lesbians and Gay Men: Chemical Dependency Treatment Issues*. Binghamton, NY: Harrington Park Press.

ETHNIC, RACIAL, AND CULTURAL MINORITY GROUPS

Chan CS. 1987. Asian lesbians: Psychological issues in the "coming out" process. *Asian American Psychological Association Journal* 12:16–18.

Chan CS. 1989. Issues of identity development among Asian American lesbians and gay men. *Journal of Couseling and Development* 68(1):16–20.

Chan CS. 1992. Cultural considerations in counseling Asian American lesbians and gay men. In: Dworkin S, Gutierrez F, eds. *Counseling Gay Men and Lesbians*. Alexandria, VA: American Association for Counseling and Development. Pp. 115–124.

Chan CS. 1993. Issues of identity development among Asian-American lesbians and gay men. In: Garnets LD, Kimmel DC, eds. *Psychosocial Perspectives on Lesbian and Gay Male Experiences. Between Men—Between Women: Lesbian and Gay Studies*. New York: Columbia University Press. Pp. 376–387.

Chan CS. 1995. Issues of sexual identity in an ethnic minority: The case of Chinese American lesbians, gay men, and bisexual people. In: D'Augelli AR, Patterson CJ, eds. *Lesbian, Gay, and Bisexual Identities over the Lifespan: Psychological Perspectives*. New York: Oxford University Press. Pp. 87–101.

Cochran SD, Mays VM. 1988. Disclosure of sexual preference to physicians by black lesbian and bisexual women. *Western Journal of Medicine* 149(5):616–619.

Cochran SC, Mays VM. 1994. Depressive distress among homosexually active African American men and women. *American Journal of Psychiatry* 151(4):524–529.

Comas DL, Greene B, ed. 1994. *Women of Color: Integrating Ethnic and Gender Identities in Psychotherapy*. Washington, DC: Transcultural Mental Health Institute.

Espin O. 1987. Issues of identity in the psychology of Latina lesbians: Exploration and challenges. In: Boston Lesbian Psychologies Collective, eds. *Lesbian Psychologies*. Urbana, IL: University of Illinois Press. Pp. 33–51.

Gomez J, Smith B. 1990. Taking the home out of homophobia: Black lesbian health. In: White EC, ed. *The Black Women's Health Book: Speaking for Ourselves*. Seattle, WA: Seal Press. Pp. 198–213.

Greene B. 1986. When the therapist is white and the patient is black: Considerations for psychotherapy in the feminist heterosexual and homosexual communities. Special Issue: The dynamics of feminist therapy. *Women and Therapy* 5(2–3):41–65.

Greene B. 1994. Ethnic-minority lesbians and gay men: Mental health and treatment issues. *Journal of Consulting and Clinical Psychology* 62(2):243–251.

Greene B. 1994. Lesbian women of color: Triple jeopardy. In: Comas-Díaz L, Greene B, eds. *Women of Color: Integrating Ethnic and Gender Identities in Psychotherapy.* New York: Guilford Press. Pp. 389–427.

Greene B. 1996. African American lesbians: Triple jeopardy. In: Brown-Collins A, ed. *The Psychology of Afican American Women.* New York: Guilford Press.

Greene B. 1996. African-American women: Considering diverse identities and societal barriers in psychotherapy. *Annals of the New York Academy of Sciences* 789:191–209.

Greene B. 1996c. Lesbians and gay men of color: The legacy of ethnosexual mythologies in heterosexism. In: Rothblum ED, Bond LA, eds. *Preventing Heterosexism and Homophobia.* Thousand Oaks, CA: Sage Publications. Pp. 59–70.

Greene B, Boyd-Franklin N. 1996. African American lesbians: Issues in couples therapy. In: Laird J, Green R-J, eds. *Lesbians and Gays in Couples and Families: A Handbook for Therapists.* San Francisco, CA: Jossey-Bass. Pp. 251–271.

Gutierrez F, Dworkin S. 1992. Gay, lesbian, and African American: Managing the integration of identities. In: Dworkin S, Gutierrez F, eds. *Counseling Gay Men and Lesbians: Journey to the End of the Rainbow.* Alexandria, VA: American Association for Counseling and Development. Pp. 141–156.

Hidalgo H, ed. 1995. *Lesbians of Color: Social and Human Services.* New York: Harrington Park Press/Haworth Press.

Hidalgo H. 1995. The norms of conduct in social service agencies: A threat to the mental health of Puerto Rican lesbians. In: Hidalgo H, ed. *Lesbians of Color: Social and Human Services.* New York. Harrington Park Press/Haworth Press: Pp. 23–41.

Jones BE, Hill MJ. 1996. African American lesbians, gay men, and bisexuals. In: Cabaj RP, Stein TS, eds. *Textbook of Homosexuality and Mental Health.* Washington, DC: American Psychiatric Press.

Kanuha V. 1990. Compounding the triple jeopardy: Battering in lesbian of color relationships. Special Issue: Diversity and complexity in feminist therapy: I. *Women and Therapy* 9(1–2):169–184.

Krieger N, Sidney S. 1997. Prevalence and health implications of anti-gay discrimination: A study of black and white women and men in the CARDIA cohort. *International Journal of Health Services* 27(1):157–176.

Leifer C, Young EW. 1997. Homeless lesbians: Psychology of the hidden, the disenfranchised, and the forgotten. *Journal of Psychosocial Nursing and Mental Health Services* 35(10):28–33.

Liu P, Chan CS. 1996. Lesbian, gay, and bisexual Asian Americans and their families. In: Laird J, Green R-J, eds. *Lesbians and Gays in Couples and Families: A Handbook for Therapists.* San Francisco: Jossey-Bass. Pp. 137–152.

Mays VM, Cochran SD. 1988. The black women's relationship project: A national survey of black lesbians. In: Shernoff M, Scott W, eds. *The Sourcebook on Lesbian/Gay Health Care,* 2nd Edition. Washington, DC: National Gay and Lesbian Health Foundation. Pp. 54–62.

Mays VM, Cochran SD, Rhue S. 1993. The impact of perceived discrimination on the intimate relationships of black lesbians. *Journal of Homosexuality* 25(4):1–14.

Mays VM, Beckman LJ, Oranchak E, Harper B. 1994. Perceived social support for help-seeking behaviors of black heterosexual and homosexually active women alcoholics. *Psychology of Addictive Behaviors* 8(4):235–242.

Morales E. 1992. Latino gays and Latina lesbians. In: Dworkin S, Gutierrez F, eds. *Counseling Gay Men and Lesbians: Journey to the End of the Rainbow*. Alexandria, VA: American Association for Counseling and Development. Pp. 125–139.

Morales E. 1996. Gender roles among Latino gay and bisexual men: Implications for family and couple relationships. In: Laird J, Green R-J, eds. *Lesbians and Gays in Couples and Families: A Handbook for Therapists*. San Francisco: Jossey-Bass. Pp. 272–297.

Nakajima GA, Chan YH, Lee K. 1996. Mental health issues for gay and lesbian Asian Americans. In: Cabaj RP, Stein TS, eds. *Textbook of Homosexuality and Mental Health*. Washington, DC: American Psychiatric Press. Pp. 563–581.

National Asian Women's Health Organization. 1996. *Asian Lesbian and Bisexual Women's Health Project: A San Francisco Bay Area Needs Assessment*. San Francisco: National Asian Women's Health Organization (NAWHO).

Savin-Williams RC. 1996a. Ethnic- and sexual-minority youth. In: Savin-Williams RC, Cohen KM, eds. *The Lives of Lesbians, Gays, and Bisexuals: Children to Adults*. Fort Worth, TX: Harcourt Brace College Publishers. Pp. 152–165.

Stevens PE. 1992. Health Care Experiences of a Racially and Economically Diverse Group of Lesbians: A Feminist Narrative Study. A dissertation, University of California at San Francisco.

Sullivan G, Leong L, Wai T, eds. 1995. *Gays and Lesbians in Asia and the Pacific: Social and Human Services*. New York: Harrington Park Press/Haworth Press.

Tafoya T, Rowell R. 1988. Counseling Native American lesbians and gays. In: Shernoff M, Scott WA, eds. *The Sourcebook on Lesbian/Gay Health Care*. Washington, DC: National Lesbian and Gay Health Foundation. Pp. 63–67.

Tremble B, Schneider M, Appathurai C. 1989. Growing up gay or lesbian in a multicultural context. *Journal of Homosexuality* 17(3–4):253–267.

Weinrich J, Williams WL. 1991. Strange customs, familiar lives: Homosexuality in other cultures. In: Gonsiorek J, Weinrich J, eds. *Homosexuality: Research Findings for Public Policy*. Newbury Park, CA: Sage Publications. Pp. 44–59.

Whitam FL, Daskalos C, Sobolewski CG, Padilla P. 1998. The emergence of lesbian sexuality and identity cross-culturally: Brazil, Peru, the Philippines, and the United States. *Archives of Sexual Behavior* 27(1):31–56.

FAMILY

Baptiste DA, Jr. 1987. Psychotherapy with gay/lesbian couples and their children in "step-families": A challenge for marriage and family therapists. *Journal of Homosexuality* 14(1–2):223–238.

Bozett FW, ed. 1987. *Gay and Lesbian Parents*. New York: Praeger Publishers.

Brewaeys A, van Ball EV. 1997. Lesbian motherhood: The impact on child development and family functioning. *Journal of Psychosomatic Obstetrics and Gynaecology* 18:116.

Brewaeys A, Ponjaert I, van Ball EV, Golombok S. 1997. Donor insemination: Child development and family functioning in lesbian mother families. *Human Reproduction* 12:1349–1359.

Brewaeys A, Ponjaert-Kristoffersen I, Van Steirteghem AC, Devroey P. 1993. Children from anonymous donors: An inquiry into homosexual and heterosexual parents' attitudes. *Journal of Psychosomatic Obstetrics and Gynaecology* 14(Suppl):23–35.

Cameron P, Cameron K. 1997. Did the APA misrepresent the scientific literature to courts in support of homosexual custody? *Journal of Psychology* 131(3):313–332.

Crawford S. 1987. Lesbian families: Psychosocial stress and the family-building process. In: Boston Lesbian Psychologies Collective, eds. *Lesbian Psychologies.* Chicago, IL: University of Illinois Press. Pp. 195–214.

Dahlheimer D, Feigal J. 1994. Community as family: The multiple-family contexts of gay and lesbian clients. In: Huber CH, ed. *Transitioning from Individual to Family Counseling. The Family Psychology and Counseling Series,* No. 2. Alexandria, VA: American Counseling Association. Pp. 63–74.

Falk P. 1993. Lesbian mothers: Psychosocial assumptions and family law. In: Garnets LD, Kimmel DC, eds. *Psychological Perspectives on Lesbian and Gay Male Experience.* New York: Columbia University Press. Pp. 420–436.

Gartrell N, Hamilton J, Banks A, Mosbacher D, Reed N, Sparks C, Bishop H. 1996. The national lesbian family study: 1. Interviews with prospective mothers. *American Journal of Orthopsychiatry* 66(2):272–281.

Gold MA, Perrin EC, Futterman D, Friedman SB. 1994. Children of gay or lesbian parents. *Pediatrics in Review* 15(9):354–358.

Golombok S, Tasker F. 1994. Donor insemination for single heterosexual and lesbian women: Issues concerning the welfare of the child. *Human Reproduction* 9(11):1972–1976.

Golombok S, Tasker F, Murray C. 1997. Children raised in fatherless families from infancy: Family relationships and the socioemotional development of children of lesbian and single heterosexual mothers. *Journal of Child Psychology and Psychiatry* 38(7):783–791.

Gottman JS. 1989. Children of gay and lesbian parents. *Marriage and Family Review* 14:177–196.

Green GD. 1987. Lesbian mothers: Mental health considerations. In: Bozett FW, ed. *Gay and Lesbian Parents.* New York: Praeger Publishers. Pp. 188–198.

Hammer SG. 1997. Gay and lesbian parents [letter; comment]. *Pediatrics* 99(2):307–308.

Harvey SM, Carr C, Bernheine S. 1989. Lesbian mothers. Health care experiences. *Journal of Nurse Midwifery* 34(3):115–119.

Hoeffer B. 1981. Children's acquisition of sex-role behavior in lesbian-mother families. *American Journal of Orthopsychiatry* 51(3):536–544.

Kenney JW, Tash DT. 1992. Lesbian childbearing couples' dilemmas and decisions. *Health Care for Women International* 13(2):209–219.

Laird J. 1993. Lesbian and gay families. In: Walsh F, ed. *Normal Family Processes,* 2nd Edition. New York: Guilford Press. Pp. 282–328.

Laird J. 1994. Lesbian families: A cultural perspective. In: Pravder Mirkin M, ed. *Women in Context: Toward a Feminist Reconstruction of Psychotherapy.* New York: Guilford Press. Pp. 118–148.

Litwin J. 1993. The lesbian childbearing couple: A case report [letter; comment]. *Birth* 20(3):168.

McNeill KF, Rienzi BM, Kposowa A. 1998. Families and parenting: A comparison of lesbian and heterosexual mothers. *Psychological Reports* 82(1):59–62.

Mitchell V. 1996. Two moms: Contribution of the planned lesbian family to the deconstruction of gendered parenting. In: Laird J, Green R-J, eds. *Lesbians and Gays in Couples and Families: A Handbook for Therapists*. San Francisco, CA: Jossey-Bass. Pp. 343–357.

Okun BF. 1996. *Understanding Diverse Families: What Practitioners Need to Know*. New York: Guilford Press.

Patterson CJ. 1992. Children of lesbian and gay parents. *Child Development* 63:1025–1042.

Patterson CJ. 1994. Children of the lesbian baby boom: Behavioral adjustment, self-concepts, and sex-role identity. In: Greene B, Herek G, eds. *Contemporary Perspectives on Gay and Lesbian Psychology: Theory, Research, and Applications*, Vol. 1. Thousand Oaks, CA: Sage Publications. Pp. 156–175.

Patterson CJ. 1996. Contributions of lesbian and gay parents and their children to the prevention of heterosexism. In: Rothblum ED, Bond LA, eds. *Preventing Heterosexism and Homophobia. Primary Prevention of Psychopathology*, Vol. 17. Thousand Oaks, CA: Sage Publications. Pp. 184–201.

Rand C, Graham DL, Rawlings EI. 1982. Psychological health and factors the court seeks to control in lesbian mother custody trials. *Journal of Homosexuality* 8(1):27–39.

Robinson BE, Walters LH, Skeen P. 1989. Response of parents to learning that their child is homosexual and concern over AIDS: A national study. *Journal of Homosexuality* 18(1–2):59–80.

Rockney RM. 1997. Gay and lesbian parents [letter; comment]. *Pediatrics* 99(2):307; discussion 308.

Shavelson E, Biaggio MK, Cross HH, Lehman RE. 1980. Lesbian women's perceptions of their parent–child relationships. *Journal of Homosexuality* 5(3):205–215.

Steinhorn A. 1982. Lesbian mothers—The invisible minority: Role of the mental health worker. *Women and Therapy* 1(4):35–48.

Tash DT, Kenney JW. 1993. The lesbian childbearing couple: A case report [see comments]. *Birth* 20(1):36–40.

Tasker F, Golombok S. 1995. Adults raised as children in lesbian families. *American Journal of Orthopsychiatry* 65(2):203–215.

Verhulst FC, Versluis-den Bieman HO, Balmus NC. 1997. Being raised by lesbian parents or in a single-parent family is no risk factor for problem behavior, however being raised as an adopted child is. *Nederlandsch Tijdschrift Voor Geneeskunde* 141(9):414–418.

Victor SB, Fish MC. 1995. Lesbian mothers and the children: A review for school psychologists. *School Psychology Review* 24(3):456–479.

Wismont JM, Reame NE. 1989. The lesbian childbearing experience: Assessing developmental tasks. *Image—The Journal of Nursing Scholarship* 21(3):137–41.

Zeidenstein L. 1990. Gynecological and childbearing needs of lesbians. *Journal of Nurse Midwifery* 35(1):10–8.

HEALTH

Biddle BS. 1993. *Health Status Indicators for Washington Area Lesbians and Bisexual Women: A Report on the Lesbian Health Clinic's First Year.* Washington, DC: Whitman-Walker Clinic.

Bradford J, Ryan C. 1988. *The National Lesbian Health Care Survey: Final Report.* Washington, DC: National Lesbian and Gay Health Foundation.

Brand PA, Rothblum ED, Solomon LJ. 1992. A comparison of lesbians, gay men, and heterosexuals on weight and restrained eating. *International Journal of Eating Disorders* 11(3):253–259.

Buenting JA. 1992. Health life-styles of lesbian and heterosexual women. Special Issue: Lesbian health: What are the issues? *Health Care for Women International* 13(2):165–171.

Bybee D, Roeder V. 1990. *Michigan Lesbian Health Survey: Results Relevant to AIDS. A Report to the Michigan Organization for Human Rights and the Michigan Department of Public Health.* Lansing: Michigan Department of Health and Human Services.

Canadian Family Physician. 1993. A context, not a disease. Gay and lesbian health [news]. *Canadian Family Physician* 39:1801, 1803.

Chrisler JC, Hemstreet AH. 1995. The diversity of women's health needs. In: Chrisler JC, Hemstreet AH, eds. *Variations on a Theme: Diversity and the Psychology of Women.* Albany, NY: State University of New York Press. Pp. 1–28.

Council of Scientific Affairs, American Medical Association. 1996. Health care needs of gay men and lesbians in the United States. *Journal of the American Medical Association* 275(17):1354–1359.

Dan AJ, ed. 1994. *Reframing Women's Health: Multidisciplinary Research and Practice.* Thousand Oaks, CA: Sage Publications.

DeAngelis T. 1994. First data released on lesbian health. *Monitor* July.

Denenberg R. 1995. Report on lesbian health. *Women's Health Issues* 5(2):81–91.

Fogel CI, Woods NF, eds. 1995. *Women's Health Care: A Comprehensive Handbook.* Thousand Oaks, CA: Sage Publications.

Gooch S. 1989. Lesbian health issues. *Nursing Standard* 3(23):42.

Haas AP. 1994. Lesbian health issues: An overview. In: Dan AJ, ed. *Reframing Women's Health: Multidisciplinary Research and Practice.* Thousand Oaks, CA: Sage Publications. Pp. 339–356.

Health Care for Women International. 1992. Special Issue: Lesbian health: What are the issues? *Health Care for Women International* 13(2):91–237.

Johnson W. 1997. NIH commissions panel on lesbian health priorities. *Washington Blade* August 8, p. 1.

Kenyon FE. 1968. Physique and physical health of female homosexuals. *Journal of Neurology, Neurosurgery and Psychiatry* 31(5):487–489.

Krieger N, Sidney S. 1996. Blood pressure: The CARDIA study of young black and white adults. *American Journal of Public Health* 86(10):1370–1378.

Lehmann JB, Lehmann CU, Kelly PJ. 1998. Development and health care needs of lesbians. *Journal of Women's Health* 7(3):379–387.

Malterud K. 1986. Health matters in lesbian women. *Tidsskr Nor Laegeforen* 106(25):2071–2074.

Michigan Organization for Human Rights. 1991. The Michigan Lesbian Health Survey. *MOHR Special Report* August:27–29.

Moran N. 1996. Lesbian health care needs. *Canadian Family Physician* 42:879–884.

Office of Women's Health Research. 1991. *Report of the National Institutes of Health: Opportunities for Research on Women's Health.* Bethesda, MD: National Institutes of Health.

Rankow EJ. 1995. Lesbian health issues for the primary care provider. *Journal of Family Practice* 40(5):486–496.

Rankow EJ. 1995. Lesbian health issues for the primary care provider [reply]. *Journal of Family Practice* 41(3):227.

Rosser S. 1993. Ignored, overlooked, or subsumed: Research on lesbian health and health care. *National Women's Studies Association Journal* 5(2):183–203.

Ryan C, Bradford J. 1993. The National Lesbian Health Care Survey: An overview. In: Garnets LD, Kimmel DC, eds. *Psychological Perspectives on Lesbian and Gay Male Experiences. Between Men—Between Women: Lesbian and Gay Studies.* New York: Columbia University Press. Pp. 541–556.

Simkin RJ. 1991. Lesbians face unique health care problems (opinion). *Canadian Medical Association Journal* 145(12):1620–1623.

Simkin RJ. 1993. Unique health concerns of lesbians. *Canadian Journal of Ob/Gyn and Women's Health Care* 5(5):516.

Smith M, Heaton C, Seiver D. 1990. Health concerns of lesbians. *Physician Assistant* 14(1):81–92.

Stern PN, ed. 1993. *Lesbian Health: What Are the Issues?* Washington, DC: Taylor and Francis.

Stevens PE. 1992. Lesbian health care research: A review of the literature from 1970 to 1990. *Health Care for Women International* 13(2):91–120.

Stevens PE. 1993. Lesbian health care research: A review of the literature from 1970 to 1990. In: Stern P *Lesbian Health: What Are the Issues?* Washington, DC: Taylor and Francis. Pp. 1–30.

Trippet SE, Bain J. 1990. Preliminary study of lesbian health concerns. *Health Values Health Behavior, Education and Promotion* 14(6):30–36.

Trippet SE, Bain J. 1993. Physical health problems and concerns of lesbians. *Health Care for Women International* 20(2):59–70.

Tully CT. 1995. In sickness and in health: Forty years of research on lesbians. In: Tully CT, ed *Lesbian Social Services: Research Issues.* New York: Harrington Park Press/Haworth Press. Pp. 1–18.

White JC, Dull VT. 1997. Health risk factors and health-seeking behavior in lesbians. *Journal of Women's Health* 6(1):103–112.

Williams KL, Jr. 1995. Lesbian health care issues [letter; comment]. *Journal of Family Practice* 41(3):224.

HEALTH CARE SERVICES

Berger RM. 1983. Health care for lesbians and gays: What social workers should know. *Journal of Social Work and Human Sexuality* 1(3):59–73.

Cassidy MA, Hughes TL. 1997. Lesbian health: Barriers to care. In: McElmurry BJ, Parker RS, eds. *Annual Review of Women's Health,* Vol. 3. New York: National League for Nursing Press. Pp. 67–87.

Edelman D. 1986. University health services sponsoring lesbian health workshops: Implications and accessibility. *Journal of American College Health* 35(1):44–45.

Edwards S, Jr. 1994. The student health center as multicultural catalyst. *Journal of American College Health* 42(5):225–228.

Eliason MJ. 1993. Cultural diversity in nursing care: The lesbian, gay, or bisexual client. *Journal of Transcultural Nursing* 5(1):14–20.

Eliason MJ. 1996. Caring for the lesbian, gay, or bisexual patient: Issues for critical care nurses. *Critical Care Nursing Quarterly* 19(1):65–72.

Eliason MJ. 1996. *Who Cares? Institutional Barriers to Health Care for Lesbian, Gay, and Bisexual Persons.* New York: National League for Nursing Press.

Ettelbrick PL. 1996. Legal issues in health care for lesbians and gay men. In: Peterson KJ, ed. *Health Care for Lesbians and Gay Men: Confronting Homophobia and Heterosexism.* New York: Harrington Park Press/Haworth Press. Pp. 93–109.

Fletcher JL, Payne FE. 1995. Lesbian health issues for the primary care provider [letter, comment]. *Journal of Family Practice* 41(3):227.

Gambrill ED, Stein TJ, Brown CE. 1984. Social services use and need among gay/lesbian residents of the San Francisco Bay Area. *Journal of Social Work and Human Sexuality* 3(1):51–69.

Geddes VA. 1994. Lesbian expectations and experiences with family doctors. How much does the physician's sex matter to lesbians? *Canadian Family Physician* 40:908–920.

Gentry SE. 1992. Caring for lesbians in a homophobic society. *Health Care for Women International* 13(2):173–180.

Gibson G, Saunders DE. 1994. Gay patients. Context for care [see comments]. *Canadian Family Physician* 40:721–725.

Gonsiorek JC. 1981. Organizational and staff problems in gay/lesbian mental health agencies. *Journal of Homosexuality* 7(2–3):193–208.

Harrison AE. 1996. Primary care of lesbian and gay patients: Educating ourselves and our students [see comments]. *Family Medicine* 28(1):10–23.

Harrison AE, Silenzio VM. 1996. Comprehensive care of lesbian and gay patients and families. *Primary Care* 23(1):31–46.

Hitchcock JM, Wilson HS. 1992. Personal risking: Lesbian self-disclosure of sexual orientation to professional health care providers. *Nursing Research* 41(3):178–183.

Johnson SR, Guenther SM. 1987. The role of "coming out" by the lesbians in the physician–patient relationship. Special Issue: Women, power, and therapy: Issues for women. *Women and Therapy* 6(1–2):231–238.

Johnson SR, Palermo JL. 1984. Gynecologic care for the lesbian. *Clinical Obstetrics and Gynecology* 27(3):724–731.

Johnson SR, Smith EM, Guenther SM. 1987. Comparison of gynecologic health care problems between lesbians and bisexual women. A survey of 2,345 women. *Journal of Reproductive Medicine* 32(11):805–811.

Johnson SR, Guenther SM, Laube DW, Keettel WC. 1981. Factors influencing lesbian gynecologic care: A preliminary study. *American Journal of Obstetrics and Gynecology* 140(1):20–28.

Lucas VA. 1992. An investigation of the health care preferences of the lesbian population. *Health Care for Women International* 13(2):221–228.

Lynch MA. 1993. When the patient is also a lesbian. *AWHONNS Clinical Issues in Perinatal Womens Health Nursing* 4(2):196–202.

MacEwan I. 1994. Differences in assessment and treatment approaches for homosexual clients. *Drug and Alcohol Review* 13(1):57–62.

Mapou RL. 1990. Traumatic brain injury rehabilitation with gay and lesbian individuals. *Journal of Head Trauma Rehabilitation* 5(2):67–72.

Perkins RE. 1996. Women, lesbians and community care. In: Abel K, Buszewicz M, Davison S, Johnson S, et al., eds. *Planning Community Mental Health Services for Women: A Multiprofessional Handbook*. London: Routledge. Pp. 79–93.

Perrin EC, Kulkin H. 1996. Pediatric care for children whose parents are gay or lesbian [see comments]. *Pediatrics* 97(5):629–635.

Potter S. 1984. Social work, traditional health care systems and lesbian invisibility. Special Issue: Feminist perspectives on social work and human sexuality. *Journal of Social Work and Human Sexuality* 3(2–3):59–68.

Rankow EJ. 1997. Primary medical care of the gay or lesbian patient. *North Carolina Medical Journal* 58(2):92–96.

Roberts SJ, Sorensen L. 1995. Lesbian health care: A review and recommendations for health promotion in primary care settings. *Nurse Practitioner* 20(6):42–47.

Robertson MM. 1992. Lesbians as an invisible minority in the health services arena. *Health Care for Women International* 13(2):155–163.

Robertson MM. 1993. Lesbians as an invisible minority in the health services arena. In: Stern P, ed. *Lesbian Health: What Are the issues?* Washington, DC: Taylor and Francis. Pp. 65–73.

Stevens PE. 1993. Marginalized women's access to health care: A feminist narrative style. *Advances in Nursing Science* 5(4):39–56.

Stevens PE. 1995. Structural and interpersonal impact of heterosexual assumptions on lesbian health care clients. *Nursing Research* 44(1):25–30.

Stevens PE. 1996. Lesbians and doctors: Experiences of solidarity and domination in health care settings. *Gender and Society* 10(1):24–41.

Stevens PE, Hall JM. 1988. Stigma, health beliefs and experiences with health care in lesbian women. *Image—Journal of Nursing Scholarship* 20(2):69–73.

Stine K. 1997. Health care for lesbians. Issues and influences. *Advances in Nursing Practice* 5(11):60–62.

Stone BH. 1997. A visit to your health care provider. *Journal of the Gay and Lesbian Medical Association* 1(1):49–50.

Temple-Smith M, Hammond J, Pyett P, Presswell N. 1996. Barriers to sexual history taking in general practice. *Australian Family Physician* 25(9 Suppl 2):S71–S74.

Trippet SE, Bain J. 1992. Reasons American lesbians fail to seek traditional health care. Special Issue: Lesbian health: What are the issues? *Health Care for Women International* 13(2):145–153.

Trippet SE, Bain J. 1993. Reasons American lesbians fail to seek traditional health care. In: Stern PN, ed. *Lesbian Health: What Are the Issues?* Washington, DC: Taylor and Francis. Pp. 55–63.

White J, Levinson W. 1993. Primary care of lesbian patients. *Journal of General Internal Medicine* 8(1):41–47.

White JC, Levinson W. 1995. Lesbian health care. What a primary care physician needs to know. *Western Journal of Medicine* 162(5):463–466.

Whyte J, Capaldini L. 1980. Treating the lesbian or gay patient. *Delaware Medical Journal* 52(5):271–277.

HIV/AIDS

Bevier PJ, CMA, HRT, Castro KG. 1995. Women at a sexually transmitted disease clinic who reported same-sex contact: Their HIV seroprevalence and risk behaviors. *American Journal of Public Health* 85(10):1366–1371.

Broun S. 1996. Clinical and psychosocial issues of women with HIV/AIDS. In: O'Leary A, Jemmott LS, eds. *Women and AIDS: Coping and Care. AIDS Prevention and Mental Health.* New York: Plenum Press. Pp. 151–166.

Centers for Disease Control and Prevention. 1995. *Report on Lesbian HIV Issues.* Atlanta, GA: Centers for Disease Control and Prevention.

Centers for Disease Control and Prevention. 1996. *HIV/AIDS and Women Who Have Sex with Women.* Rockville, MD: CDC National AIDS Clearinghouse.

Chu SY, Buehler JW, Fleming PL, Berkelman RL. 1990. Epidemiology of reported cases of AIDS in lesbians, United States 1980–89. *American Journal of Public Health* 80(11):1380–1381.

Chu SY, Hammett TA, Buehler JW. 1992. Update: Epidemiology of reported cases of AIDS in women who report sex only with other women, United States, 1980–1991 [letter]. *AIDS* 6:518–519.

Cochran SD, Bybee D, Gage S, Mays VM. 1996. Prevalence of HIV-related self-reported sexual behaviors, sexually transmitted diseases, and problems with drugs and alcohol in 3 large surveys of lesbian and bisexual women: A look into a segment of the community. *Women's Health Research on Gender, Behavior, and Policy* 2(1–2):11–33.

Cohen H, Marmor M, Wolfe H, Ribble D. 1993. Risk assessment of HIV transmission among lesbians [letter]. *Journal of Acquired Immune Deficiency Syndrome* 6(10):1173–1174.

Cranston K. 1991. HIV education for gay, lesbian, and bisexual youth: Personal risk, personal power, and the community of conscience. Special Issue: Coming out of the classroom closet: Gay and lesbian students, teachers, and curricula. *Journal of Homosexuality* 22(3–4):247–259.

Deren S, Goldstein M, Williams M, Stark M, Estrada A, Friedman SR, Young RM. 1996. Sexual orientation, HIV risk behavior, and serostatus in a multisite sample of drug-injecting and crack-using women. *Women's Health: Research on Gender, Behavior, and Policy* 2(1–2):35–47.

Einhorn L, Polgar M. 1994. HIV-risk behavior among lesbians and bisexual women. *AIDS Education and Prevention* 6(6):514–523.

Fortney JT, Kudler H, Mann ES. 1997. Gays, lesbians, HIV infection, and admission to medical school. A physicians' roundtable. *North Carolina Medical Journal* 58(2):126–128.

Friedman SR, Jose B, Deren S, Des Jarlis DC, Neaigus A, National AIDS Research Consortium. 1995. Risk factors for HIV seroconversion among out-of-treatment drug injectors in high- and low-seroprevalence cities. *American Journal of Epidemiology,* 142(8):864–874.

Friedman SR. 1998. Women drug injectors who have sex with women: Heightened risk and unknown reasons suggest the need for further research. *Newsletter of the International AIDS Society* 11:12–13.

Gay and Lesbian Medical Association. 1997. *HIV-Positive Health Care Workers: The Need for Revisions in CDC Guidelines.* San Francisco, CA: Gay and Lesbian Medical Association.

Gómez CA. 1994. Lesbians at risk for HIV: An unresolved debate. In: Greene B, Herek GM eds. *Psychosocial Perspectives on Lesbian and Gay Issues,* Vol. 1: *Lesbian and Gay Psychology: Theory, Research, and Clinical Applications.* Thousand Oaks, CA: Sage Publications.

Gómez CA, Garcia DR, Kegebein VJ, Shade SB, Hernandez SR. 1996. Sexual identity versus sexual behavior: Implications for HIV prevention strategies for women who have sex with women. *Women's Health: Research on Gender, Behavior, and Policy* 2(1–2):91–109.

Harris NV, Thiede H, McGough JP, Gordon D. 1993. Risk factors for HIV infection among injection drug users: Results of blinded surveys in drug treatment centers, King County, Washington 1988–1991. *Journal of Acquired Immune Deficiency Syndrome* 6(11):1275–1282.

Hunter J, Alexander P. 1997. Women who sleep with women. In: Long LD, Ankrah EM, eds. *AIDS and Women's Experience: Emerging Political Agendas.* New York: Columbia University Press.

Hunter J, Schaecher R. 1994. AIDS prevention for lesbian, gay, and bisexual adolescents. Special Issue: HIV/AIDS. *Families in Society* 75(6):346–354.

Jones A, Billy S. 1990. Sexual minority needle users. In: Leukefeld CG, Battjes RJ, Amsel Z, eds. *AIDS and Intravenous Drug Use: Future Directions for Community-Based Prevention Research.* NIDA Research Monograph 93. Rockville, MD: National Institute on Drug Abuse. Pp. 108–119.

Jose B, Friedman SR, Neaigus A, Curtis R, Grund JPC, Goldstein M, Ward T, Des Jarlais DC. 1993. Syringe-mediated drug-sharing (backloading): A new risk factor for HIV among injecting drug users. *AIDS* 7:1653–1660.

Kennedy MB, Scarlett MI, Duerr AC, Chu SY. 1995. Assessing HIV risk among women who have sex with women: Scientific and communication issues. *Journal of the American Medical Womens Association* 50(3–4):103–107.

Kral AH, Lorvick J, Bluthenthal RN, Watters JK. 1997. HIV risk profile of drug-using women who have sex with women in 19 United States cities. *Journal of Acquired Immune Deficiency Syndromes and Human Retrovirology* 16(3):211–217.

Lemp GF, Jones M, Kellogg TA, Nieri GN, et al. 1995. HIV seroprevalence and risk behaviors among lesbians and bisexual women in San Francisco and Berkeley, California. *American Journal of Public Health* 85(11):1549–1552.

Lloyd GA, Kuszelewicz MA, eds. 1995. *HIV Disease: Lesbians, Gays and the Social Services.* New York: Harrington Park Press/Haworth Press.

Magura S, O'Day J, Rosenblum A. 1992. Women usually take care of their girlfriends: Bisexuality and HIV risk among female intravenous drug users. *Journal of Drug Issues* 22(1):179–190.

Marrazzo JM, Stine K, Handsfield HH, Kiviat NB, Koutsky LA. 1996. HIV-related risk behavior in a community-based sample of women who have sex with women. *XI International Conference on AIDS/HIV*, Vancouver, Canada, July 7–12.

Mays VM. 1996. Are lesbians at risk for HIV infection? *Women's Health: Research on Gender, Behavior, and Policy* 2(1–2):1–9.

Mays VM, Cochran SD, Pies C, Chu SY, Ehrhardt AA. 1996. The risk of HIV infection for lesbians and other women who have sex with women: Implications for HIV research, prevention, policy, and services. *Women's Health: Research on Gender, Behavior, and Policy* 2(1–2):119–139.

Morrow KM. 1995. Lesbian women and HIV/AIDS: An appeal for inclusion. In: O'Leary A, Sweet Jemmott L, eds. *Women at Risk: Issues in the Primary Prevention of AIDS. AIDS Prevention and Mental Health.* New York: Plenum Press. Pp. 237–256.

Morrow KM, Fuqua RW, Meinhold PM. 1994. Self-reported HIV risk behaviors and serostatus in lesbian and bisexual women. *Psychosocial and Behavioral Factors in Women's Health: Creating an Agenda for the 21st Century.* Washington, DC: American Psychological Association.

National Minority AIDS Council. 1997. The Consumer Survey: A project of the Philadelphia EMA HIV Commission—Results from multivariate analysis. 1997 U.S. Conference on AIDS, Miami Beach, FL, September. Washington, DC: National Minority AIDS Council.

National Research Council. 1989. *AIDS: Sexual Behavior and Intravenous Drug Use.* Washington, DC: National Academy Press.

Norman AD, Perry MJ, Stevenson LY, Kelly JA, Roffman RA. 1996. Lesbian and bisexual women in small cities—At risk for HIV? HIV Prevention Community Collaborative. *Public Health Reports* 111(4):347–352.

O'Leary A, Jemmott LS, eds. 1995. *Women at Risk: Issues in the Primary Prevention of AIDS.* New York: Plenum Press.

Perry S, Jacobsberg L, Fogel K. 1989. Orogenital transmission of human immuno-deficiency virus. *Annals of Internal Medicine* 111(11):951–952.

Petersen L, Doll L, White C, Chu S. 1992. No evidence of female-to-female transmission among 960,000 female blood donors. *Journal of Acquired Immune Deficiency Syndrome* 5:853–855.

Raiteri R. 1994. Lesbian sex no risk for HIV transmission. *Nursing Standard* 8(45):17.

Raiteri R, Fora R, Sinicco A. 1994. HIV risk found 'non existent' among lesbians. *Nursing Times* 90(31):10–11.

Raiteri R, Fora R, Sinicco A. 1994. No HIV-1 transmission through lesbian sex. *Lancet* 344(8917):270.

Raiteri R, Fora R, Gioannini P, Russo R, Lucchini A, Terzi MG, Giacobbi D, Sinicco A. 1994. Seroprevalence, risk factors and attitude to HIV-1 in a representative sample of lesbians in Turin. *Genitourinary Medicine* 70(3):200–205.

Raiteri R, Baussano I, Giobbia M, Fora R, Sinicco A. 1998. Lesbian sex and risk of HIV transmission [letter]. *AIDS* 12(4):450–451.

Rankow EJ, Blackman D, Carannante T. 1994. *Lesbian AIDS Project: Bibliography of Resources Relevant to Lesbians and HIV/AIDS*. New York: Gay Men's Health Crisis.

Reynolds G. 1994. HIV and lesbian sex. *Lancet* 344(8921):544–545.

Stevens PE. 1993b. Lesbians and HIV: Clinical, research, and policy issues. *American Journal of Orthopsychiatry* 63(2):289–294.

Stevens PE. 1994. HIV prevention education for lesbians and bisexual women: A cultural analysis of a community intervention. *Social Science and Medicine* 39(11):1565–1578.

Stuntzner-Gibson D. 1991. Women and HIV disease: An emerging social crisis. *Social Work* 36(1):22–28.

Wang J, Rodes A, Blanch C, Casabona J. 1997. HIV testing history among gay/bisexual men recruited in Barcelona: Evidence of high levels of risk behavior among self-reported HIV+ men. *Social Science and Medicine* 44(4):469–477.

White JC. 1997. HIV risk assessment and prevention among lesbians and women who have sex with women: Practical information for clinicians. *Health Care for Women International* 18(2):1549–1552.

White JC. 1997. HIV risk assessment and prevention in lesbians and women who have sex with women: Practical information for clinicians. *Health Care for Women International* 18(2):127–138.

Whyte K. 1992. A community in crisis: Will mental health services respond to AIDS? *Canada's Mental Health* 40(4):2–5.

MENTAL HEALTH

Alexander CJ, ed. 1996. *Gay and Lesbian Mental Health: A Sourcebook for Practitioners*. New York: Harrington Park Press/Haworth Press.

Anderson MK, Mavis BE. 1996. Sources of coming out self-efficacy for lesbians. *Journal of Homosexuality* 32(2):37–52.

Atkinson DR, Hackett G. 1995. *Counseling Diverse Populations*. Dubuque, IA: Brown and Benchmark.

Ball S. 1994. A group model for gay and lesbian clients with chronic mental illness. *Social Work* 39(1):109–115.

Banks A, Gartrell NK. 1996. Lesbians in the medical setting. In: Cabaj RP, Stein TS, eds. *Textbook of Homosexuality and Mental Health*. Washington, DC: American Psychiatric Press. Pp. 659–671.

Baron J. 1996. Some issues in psychotherapy with gay and lesbian clients. *Psychotherapy* 33(4):611–616.

Baumrind D. 1995. Commentary on sexual orientation: Research and social policy implications. Special Issue: Sexual orientation and human development. *Developmental Psychology* 31(1):130–136.

Beren S, Hayden H, Wilfley D, Grilo C. 1996. The influence of sexual orientation on body dissatisfaction in adult men and women. *International Journal of Eating Disorders* 20(2):135–141.

Bernstein GS, Miller ME. 1996. Behavior therapy with lesbian and gay individuals. *Progress in Behavior Modification* 30:123–136.

Betz NE, Fitzgerald LF. 1993. Individuality and diversity: Theory and research in counseling psychology. *Annual Review of Psychology* 44: 343–381.

Bradford J, Plumb M, White J, Ryan C. 1994. Information transfer strategies to support lesbian research. *Psychological and Behavioral Factors in Women's Health: Creating an Agenda for the 21st Century—Conference Proceedings,* Washington, DC, May. Washington, DC: American Psychological Association.

Bradford J, Ryan C, Rothblum ED. 1994. National Lesbian Health Care Survey: Implications for mental health care. *Journal of Consulting and Clinical Psychology* 62(2):228–242.

Brown LS. 1996. Ethical concerns with sexual minority patients. In: Cabaj RP, Stein TS, eds. *Textbook of Homosexuality and Mental Health.* Washington, DC: American Psychiatric Press. Pp. 897–916.

Cabaj RP. 1996. Gay, lesbian, and bisexual mental health professionals and their colleagues. In: Cabaj RP, Stein TS, eds. *Textbook of Homosexuality and Mental Health.* Washington, DC: American Psychiatric Press. Pp. 33–39.

Cabaj RP. 1996. Sexual orientation of the therapist. In: Cabaj RP, Stein TS, eds. *Textbook of Homosexuality and Mental Health.* Washington, DC: American Psychiatric Press. Pp. 513–524.

Cabaj RP, Stein TS, eds. 1996. *Textbook of Homosexuality and Mental Health.* Washington, DC: American Psychiatric Press.

Casas JM, Brady S, Ponterotto JG. 1983. Sexual preference biases in counseling: An information processing approach. *Journal of Counseling Psychology* 30(2):139–145.

Cass V. 1996. Sexual orientation identity formation: A Western phenomenon. In: Cabaj RP, Stein TS, eds. *Textbook of Homosexuality and Mental Health.* Washington, DC: American Psychiatric Press. Pp. 227–251.

Chrisler JC, Hemstreet AH, eds. 1995. *Variations on a Theme: Diversity and the Psychology of Women.* Albany, NY: State University of New York Press.

Christie D, Young M. 1986. Self-concept of lesbian and heterosexual women. *Psychological Reports* 59:1279–1282.

Cohler BJ, Galatzer LR. 1996. Self psychology and homosexuality: Sexual orientation and maintenance of personal integrity. In: Cabaj RP, Stein TS, eds. *Textbook of Homosexuality and Mental Health.* Washington, DC: American Psychiatric Press. Pp. 207–223.

Committee on Professional Standards. 1986. Casebook for providers of psychological services. *American Psychologist* 41(6):688–693.

Crawford S. 1988. Cultural context as a factor in the expansion of therapeutic conversation with lesbian families. *Journal of Strategic and Systemic Therapies* 7(3):2–10.

D'Augelli AR. 1993. Preventing mental health problems among lesbian and gay college students. *Journal of Primary Prevention* 13(4):245–261.

D'Augelli AR, Garnets LD. 1995. Lesbian, gay, and bisexual communities. In: D'Augelli AR, Patterson CJ, eds. *Lesbian, Gay, and Bisexual Identities over the Lifespan: Psychological Perspectives.* New York: Oxford University Press. Pp. 293–320.

DeAngelis T. 1994. APA, NIMH discuss gay, lesbian issues. *Monitor* July.

Deevey S, Wall LJ. 1992. How do lesbian women develop serenity? Special Issue: Lesbian health: What are the issues? *Health Care for Women International* 13 (2):199–208.

Dickenson D, Johnson M, eds. 1993. *Death, Dying and Bereavement.* London: Sage Publications.

Dorrell B. 1990. Being there: A support network of lesbian women. *Journal of Homosexuality* 20(3–4):89–98.

Falco KL. 1991. *Psychotherapy with Lesbian Clients: Theory Into Practice*. New York: Brunner/Mazel, Inc.

Falco KL. 1995. Therapy with lesbians: The essentials. *Psychotherapy in Private Practice* 13(4):69–83.

Ferguson KD, Finkler DC. 1978. An involvement and overtness measure for lesbians: Its development and relation to anxiety and social zeitgeist. *Archives of Sexual Behavior* 7(3):211–227.

Garnets LD, Kimmel DC, eds. 1993. *Psychological Perspectives on Lesbian and Gay Male Experiences*. New York: Columbia University Press.

Garnets L, Hancock KA, Cochran SD, Goodchilds J, Peplau LA. 1991. Issues in psychotherapy with lesbians and gay men. A survey of psychologists. *American Psychologist* 46(9):964–972.

Garnets L, Hancock KA, Cohchran SD, Goodchilds J, Peplau LA, Sobocinski MR. 1993. Working with special populations. III: Lesbians and gay men. In: Mindell JA, ed. *in Clinical Psychology*. Dubuque, IA: Wm. C. Brown Publishers. Pp. 309–328.

Gartrell N. 1981. The lesbian as a "single" woman. *American Journal of Psychotherapy* 35(4):502–516.

Gartrell N. 1987. No: The lesbian as a "single" woman. In: Walsh MR,ed. *The Psychology of Women: Ongoing Debates*. New Haven, CT: Yale University Press. Pp. 412–420.

Gluth DR, Kiselica MS. 1994. Coming out quickly: A brief counseling approach to dealing with gay and lesbian adjustment issues. *Journal of Mental Health Counseling* 16(2):163–173.

Gonsiorek JC. 1981. Present and future directions in gay/lesbian mental health. *Journal of Homosexuality* 7(2–3):5–7.

Gonsiorek JC. 1981. The use of diagnostic concepts in working with gay and lesbian populations. Special Issue: Homosexuality and psychotherapy. *Journal of Homosexuality* 7(2–3):9–20.

Gonsiorek JC. 1993. Threat, stress, and adjustment: Mental health and the workplace for gay and lesbian individuals. In: Diamant L, ed. *Homosexual Issues in the Workplace. Series in Clinical and Community Psychology*. Washington, DC: Taylor and Francis. Pp. 243–264.

Gonsiorek JC. 1996. Mental health and sexual orientation. In: Savin-Williams R, Cohen K, eds. *The Lives of Lesbians, Gays, and Bisexuals: Children to Adults*. Fort Worth, TX: Harcourt Brace College Publishers. Pp. 462–478.

Gonsiorek JC, Rudolph JR. 1991. Homosexual identity: Coming out and other developmental events. In: Gonsiorek JC, Weinrich JD, eds. *Homosexuality: Research Implications for Public Policy*. Newbury Park, CA: Sage Publications. Pp. 161–176.

Goodrich TJ, Ellman B, Rampage C, Halstead K. 1990. The lesbian couple. In: Mirkin MP, ed. *The Social and Political Contexts of Family Therapy*. Boston, MA: Allyn & Bacon, Inc. Pp. 159–178.

Gould D. 1995. A critical examination of the notion of pathology in psychoanalysis. In: Glassgold JM, Iasenza S, eds. *Lesbians and Psychoanalysis: Revolutions in Theory and Practice*. New York: Free Press. Pp. 3–17.

Green GD. 1990. Is separation really so great? Special Issue: Diversity and complexity in feminist therapy: I. *Women and Therapy* 9(1-2):87–104.

Greene B, Herek GM, eds. 1994. *Lesbian and Gay Psychology: Theory, Research, and Clinical Applications.* Thousand Oaks, CA: Sage Publications.

Grossman AH, Kerner MS. 1998. Self-esteem and supportiveness as predictors of emotional distress in gay male and lesbian youth. *Journal of Homosexuality* 35(2):25–39.

Haldeman DC. 1994. The practice and ethics of sexual orientation conversion therapy. *Journal of Consulting and Clinical Psychology* 62(2):221–227.

Hanley-Hackenbruck P. 1993. Working with lesbians in psychotherapy. In: Odham JM, Riba MB, Tasman A, eds. *Review of Psychiatry,* Vol. 12. Washington, DC: American Psychiatric Press, Inc. Pp. 59–83.

Heffernan K. 1994. Sexual orientation as a factor in risk for binge eating and bulimia nervosa: A review. *International Journal of Eating Disorders* 16(4):335–347.

Heffernan K. 1996. Eating disorders and weight concern among lesbians. *International Journal of Eating Disorders* 19(2):127–138.

Helfand KL. 1993. Therapeutic considerations in structuring a support group for the mentally ill gay/lesbian population. *Journal of Gay and Lesbian Psychotherapy* 2(1):65–76.

Hellman RE. 1996. Issues in the treatment of lesbian women and gay men with chronic mental illness. *Psychiatric Services* 47(10):1093–1098.

Herman E. 1995. *Psychiatry, Psychology, and Homosexuality.* New York: Chelsea House Publishers.

Hiatt D, Hargrave GE. 1994. Psychological assessment of gay and lesbian law enforcement applicants. *Journal of Personality Assessment* 63(1):80–88.

Hughes TL, Haas AP, Avery L. 1997. Mental health concerns of lesbians: Preliminary results from the Chicago Women's Health Survey. *Journal of the Gay and Lesbian Medical Association* 1(3):137–148.

Igartua KJ. 1998. Therapy with lesbian couples: The issues and the interventions. *Canadian Journal of Psychiatry* 43(4):391–396.

Jordan KM, Deluty RH. 1995. Clinical interventions by psychologists with lesbians and gay men. *Journal of Clinical Psychology* 51(3):448–456.

Jordan KM, Deluty RH. 1998. Coming out for lesbian women: Its relation to anxiety, positive affectivity, self-esteem, and social support. *Journal of Homosexuality* 35(2):41–63.

Kenyon FE. 1968. Studies in female homosexuality: Psychological test results. *Journal of Consulting and Clinical Psychology* 32(5 Pt 1):510–513.

Kertzner RM, Sved M, Krajeski J. 1996. Midlife gay men and lesbians: Adult development and mental health. Homosexuality and the mental health professions: A contemporary history. In: Cabaj RP, Stein TS, eds. *Textbook of Homosexuality and Mental Health.* Washington, DC: American Psychiatric Press. Pp. 17–31.

Kessler RC, McGonagle KA, Zhao S, Nelson CB, Hughes M, Eshleman S, Wittchen H-U, Kendler KS. 1994. Lifetime and 12-month prevalence of DSM-III-R psychiatric disorders in the United States: Results from the National Comorbidity Survey. *Archives of General Psychiatry* 51:8–19.

Krajeski J. 1996. Homosexuality and the mental health professions: A contemporary history. In: Cabaj RP, Stein TS, eds. *Textbook of Homosexuality and Mental Health*. Washington, DC: American Psychiatric Press. Pp. 17–31.

Laird J, Green R-J, eds. 1996. *Lesbians and Gays in Couples and Families: A Handbook for Therapists*. San Francisco, CA: Jossey-Bass.

Leavy RL, Adams EM. 1986. Feminism as a correlate of self-esteem, self-acceptance, and social support among lesbians. *Psychology of Women Quarterly* 10(4):321–326.

Leeder E. 1996. Reflections of a midlife lesbian feminist therapist. In: Davis ND, Cole E, Rothblum ED, eds. *Lesbian Therapists and Their Therapy: From Both Sides of the Couch*. New York: Harrington Park Press/Haworth Press. Pp. 47–60.

Leiblum SR. 1997. *Infertility: Psychological Issues and Counseling Strategies*. New York: John Wiley and Sons.

Levine H. 1997. A further exploration of the lesbian identity development process and its measurement. *Journal of Homosexuality* 34(2):67–78.

Marmor J. 1996. Nongay therapists working with gay men and lesbians: A personal reflection. In: Cabaj RP, Stein TS, eds. *Textbook of Homosexuality and Mental Health*. Washington, DC: American Psychiatric Press. Pp. 539–545.

Masbaum MR. 1997. The relationship between childhood sexual abuse and substance use in a psychiatric population of women. *Journal of Addictions Nursing* 9(2):50–63.

McDaniel JS, Cabaj RP, Purcell DW. 1996. Care across the spectrum of mental health settings: Working with gay, lesbian, and bisexual patients in consultation–liaison services, inpatient treatment facilities, and community outpatient mental health centers. In: Cabaj RP, Stein TS, eds. *Textbook of Homosexuality and Mental Health*. Washington, DC: American Psychiatric Press. Pp. 687–704.

Mirkin MP, ed. 1994. *Women in Context: Toward a Feminist Reconstruction of Psychotherapy*. New York: Guilford Press.

Morgan KS. 1992. Caucasian lesbians' use of psychotherapy: A matter of attitude? *Psychology of Women Quarterly* 16(1):127–130.

Morris JF. 1997. Lesbian coming out as a multidimensional process. *Journal of Homosexuality* 33(2):1–22.

Nichols M. 1995. Sexual desire disorder in a lesbian-feminist couple: The intersection of therapy and politics. In: Rosen RC, Leiblum SR, eds. *Case Studies in Sex Therapy*. New York: Guilford Press. Pp. 161–175.

Norton JL. 1995. The gay, lesbian, and bisexual populations. In: Vacc NA, DeVaney SB, Wittmer J, eds. *Experiencing and Counseling Multicultural and Diverse Populations*. 3rd Edition. Muncie, IN: Accelerated Development, Inc. Pp. 147–177.

Perkins RE. 1996. Rejecting therapy: Using our communities. In: Rothblum ED, Bond LA, eds. *Preventing Heterosexism and Homophobia. Primary Prevention of Psychopathology*, Vol. 17. Thousand Oaks, CA: Sage Publications. Pp. 71–83.

Pribor EF, Dinwiddie SH. 1992. Psychiatric correlates of incest in childhood. *American Journal of Psychiatry* 149(1):52–56.

Ritter KY, O'Neill CW. 1989. Moving through loss: The spiritual journey of gay men and lesbian women. Special Issue: Gay, lesbian, and bisexual issues in counseling. *Journal of Counseling and Development* 68(1):9–15.

Ross MW, Paulsen JA, Stalstrom OW. 1988. Homosexuality and mental health: A cross-cultural review. *Journal of Homosexuality* 15:131–152.

Roth S. 1989. Psychotherapy with lesbian couples: Individual issues, female socialization and the social context. In: McGoldrick M, Anderson CM, Walsh F, eds. *Women in Families: A Framework for Family Therapy.* New York: W.W. Norton & Co. Pp. 286–307.

Rothblum ED. 1990. Depression among lesbians: An invisible and unresearched phenomenon. *Journal of Gay and Lesbian Psychotherapy* 1(3):67–87.

Rothblum ED. 1994. "I only read about myself on bathroom walls": The need for research on the mental health of lesbians and gay men. *Journal of Consulting and Clinical Psychology* 62(2):213–220.

Sang BE. 1992. Psychotherapy with lesbians: Some observations and tentative generalizations. In: Dynes WR, Donaldson S, eds. *Homosexuality and Psychology, Psychiatry, and Counseling. Studies in Homosexuality,* Vol. 11. New York: Garland Publishing. Pp. 260–269.

Siever MD. 1994. Sexual orientation and gender as factors in socioculturally acquired vulnerability to body dissatisfaction and eating disorders. *Journal of Consulting and Clinical Psychology* 62(2):252–260.

Silberman BO, Hawkins RO, Jr. 1988. Lesbian women and gay men: Issues for counseling. In: Weinstein E, Rosen E, eds. *Sexuality Counseling: Issues and Implications.* Pacific Grove, CA: Brooks/Cole Publishing. Pp. 101–113.

Socarides CW. 1987. Yes: Psychoanalytic perspectives on female homosexuality: A discussion of "The lesbian as a 'single' woman." In: Walsh M, ed. *The Psychology of Women: Ongoing Debates.* New Haven, CT: Yale University Press. Pp. 421–426.

Sorensen L, Roberts SJ. 1997. Lesbian uses of and satisfaction with mental health services: Results from Boston Lesbian Health Project. *Journal of Homosexuality* 33(1):35–49.

Stein TS. 1996. The essentialist/social constructionist debate about homosexuality and its relevance for psychotherapy. In: Cabaj RP, Stien TS, eds. *Textbook of Homosexuality and Mental Health.* Washington, DC: American Psychiatric Press. Pp. 83–99.

Stephany TM. 1992. Promoting mental health. Lesbian nurse support groups [see comments]. *Journal of Psychosocial Nursing and Mental Health Services* 30(2):35–38.

Stone GL, ed. 1991. Special Issues: Counseling lesbian women and gay men. *The Counseling Psychologist* 19:155–248.

Trippet SE. 1994. Lesbians' mental health concerns. *Health Care for Women International* 15(4):317–323.

Unterberger GL. 1993. Counseling lesbians: A feminist perspective. In: Wicks RJ, Parsons RD, eds. *Clinical Handbook of Pastoral Counseling,* Vol. 2: *Studies in Pastoral Psychology, Theology, and Spirituality.* New York: Springer Publishing. Pp. 73–86.

Wayment HA, Peplau LA. 1995. Social support and well-being among lesbian and heterosexual women: A structural modeling. *Personality and Social Psychology Bulletin* 21(11):1189–1199.

Woodman NJ. 1989. Mental health issues of relevance to lesbian women and gay men. *Journal of Gay and Lesbian Psychotherapy* 1(1):53–63.

METHODOLOGY

Boruch RF, Cecil JS. 1979. *Assuring the Confidentiality of Social Research Data.* Philadelphia: University of Pennsylvania Press.

Bradburn NM, Sudman S, Blair E, Locander W, Miles C, Singer E, Stocking C. 1979. *Improving Interview Method and Questionnaire Design.* San Francisco: Jossey-Bass.

Buhrke RA, Ben-Ezra LA, Hurley ME, Ruprecht LJ. 1992. Content analysis and methodological critique of articles concerning lesbian and gay male issues in counseling journals. *Journal of Counseling Psychology* 39(1):91–99.

Chung YB, Katayama M. 1996. Assessment of sexual orientation in lesbian/gay/bisexual studies. *Journal of Homosexuality* 30(4):49–62.

Donovan JM. 1992. Homosexual, gay, and lesbian: Defining the words and sampling the populations. *Journal of Homosexuality* 24(1–2):27–47.

Gonsiorek JC, Weinrich JD. 1991. The definition and scope of sexual orientation. In: Gonsiorek JC, Weinrich JD eds. *Homosexuality: Research Implications for Public Policy.* Newbury Park, CA: Sage Publications. Pp. 1–12.

Gonsiorek JC, Weinrich JD, eds. 1991. *Homosexuality: Research Implications for Public Policy.* Newbury Park, CA: Sage Publications.

Gonsiorek JC, Sell RL, Weinrich JD. 1995. Definition and measurement of sexual orientation. *Suicide and Life-Threatening Behavior* 25(Suppl):40–51.

Harris TR, Wilsnack RW, Klassen AD. 1994. Reliability of retrospective self-reports of alcohol consumption among women: Data from a U.S. national sample. *Journal of Studies on Alcohol* 55:309–314.

Hedblom JH, Hartman JJ. 1980. Research on lesbianism: Selected effects of time, geographical location, and data collection technique. *Archives of Sexual Behavior* 9(3):217–234.

Herek GM, Kimmel DC, Amaro H, Melton GB. 1991. Avoiding heterosexual bias in psychological research. *American Psychologist* 46(9):957–963.

Jacobson S. 1995. Methodological issues in research on older lesbians. In: Tully CT, ed. *Lesbian Social Services: Research Issues.* New York: Haworth Press. Pp. 43–56.

Kalton G. 1993. Sampling considerations in research on HIV risk and illness. In: Ostrow DG, Kessler RC, eds. *Methodological Issues in AIDS Behavioral Research.* New York: Plenum Press. Pp. 53–74.

Klinger A. 1998. Resources for lesbian ethnographic research in the lavender archives. *Journal of Homosexuality* 34(3–4):205–224.

LeVay S. 1996. *Queer Science: The Use and Abuse of Research into Homosexuality.* Cambridge, MA: MIT Press.

O'Hanlan KA. 1995. Lesbians in Health Research. In: *Recruitment and Retention of Women in Clinical Studies: A Report of the Workshop Sponsored by the Office of Research on Women's Health.* Rockville, MD: Office of Research on Women's Health, National Institutes of Health. Pp. 101–104.

Platzer H, James T. 1997. Methodological issues conducting sensitive research on lesbian and gay men's experience of nursing care. *Journal of Advanced Nursing* 25(3):626–633.

Sell RL, Petrulio C. 1996. Sampling homosexuals, bisexuals, gays, and lesbians for public health research: A review of the literature from 1990 to 1992. *Journal of Homosexuality* 30(4):31–47.

Skrocki FE. Use of Focus Groups to Validate an Existing Instrument for Use with Lesbians. Unpublished master's project, University of Illinois College of Nursing.

Stevens PE. 1996. Focus groups: Collecting aggregate-level data to understand community health phenomena. *Public Health Nursing* 13(3):170–176.

Turner CF, Ku L, Rogers SM, Lindberg LD, Pleck JH, Sonenstein FL. 1998. Adolescent sexual behavior, drug use, and violence: Increased reporting with computer survey technology. *Science* 280:867–873.

Turner CF, Forsyth BH, O'Reilly J, Cooley PC, Smith TK, Rogers SM, Miller HG. In press. Automated self-interviewing and the survey measurement of sensitive behaviors. In: Couper M, et al., eds. *Computer-Assisted Survey Information Collection*. New York: Wiley and Sons.

Walsh-Bowers RT, PSJ. 1992. Researcher–participant relationships in journal reports on gay men and lesbian women. *Journal of Homosexuality* 23(4):93–112.

Woodman NJ, Tully CT, Barranti CC. 1995. Research in lesbian communities: Ethical decisions. In: Tully CT, ed. *Lesbian Social Services: Research Issues*. New York: Haworth Press. Pp. 57–66.

RELATIONSHIPS

Bailey JM, Kim PY, Hills A, Linsenmeier JA. 1997. Butch, femme, or straight acting? Partner preferences of gay men and lesbians. *Journal of Personality and Social Psychology* 73(5):960–973.

Cabaj RP. 1988. Gay and lesbian couples: Lessons on human intimacy. *Psychiatric Annals* 18(1):21–25.

Caldwell MA, Peplau LA. 1984. The balance of power in lesbian relationships. *Sex Roles* 10:587–599.

Green R-J, Bettinger M, Zacks E. 1996. Are lesbian couples fused and gay male couples disengaged? Questioning gender straightjackets. In: Laird J, Green RJ, eds. *Lesbians and Gays in Couples and Families: A Handbook for Therapists*. San Francisco: Jossey-Bass. Pp. 185–230.

Healy T. 1993. A struggle for language: Patterns of self-disclosure in lesbian couples. Special Issue: Lesbians and lesbian families: Multiple reflections. *Smith College Studies in Social Work* 63(3):247–264.

Huyck MH. 1995. Marriage and close relationships of the marital kind. In: Blieszner R, Bedford VH, eds. *Handbook of Aging and the Family*. Westport, CT: Greenwood Press/Greenwood Publishing Group. Pp. 181–200.

Klinger RL, Cabaj RP. 1993. Characteristics of gay and lesbian relationships. In: Oldham JM, Riba MB, Tasman A, eds. *Review of Psychiatry,* Vol. 12. Washington, DC: American Psychiatric Press. Pp. 101–125.

Metz ME, Rosser BRS, Strapko N. 1994. Differences in conflict-resolution styles among heterosexual, gay, and lesbian couples. *Journal of Sex Research* 31(4):293–308.

Modrcin MJ, Wyers NL. 1990. Lesbian and gay couples: Where they turn when help is needed. *Journal of Gay and Lesbian Psychotherapy* 1(3):89–104.

Pearcey SM, Docherty KJ, Dabbs JM, Jr. 1996. Testosterone and sex role identification in lesbian couples. *Physiology and Behavior* 60(3):1033–1035.

Peplau LA. 1991. Lesbian and gay relationships. In: Gonsiorek JC, Weinrich JD, eds. *Homosexuality: Research Implications for Public Policy.* Newbury Park, CA: Sage Publications. Pp. 177–196.

Rolland JS. 1994. In sickness and in health: The impact of illness on couples' relationships. Special Section: Illness, health, and family therapy. *Journal of Marital and Family Therapy* 20(4):327–347.

Schneider MS. 1986. The relationships of cohabiting lesbian and heterosexual couples: A comparison. *Psychology of Women Quarterly* 10:234–239.

Simons S. 1991. Couple therapy with lesbians. In: Hooper D, Dryden W, eds. *Couple Therapy: A Handbook.* Milton Keynes, England: Open University Press. Pp. 207–216.

Smalley S. 1987. Dependency issues in lesbian relationships. *Journal of Homosexuality* 14(1–2):125–135.

Vargo S. 1987. The effect of women's socialization on lesbian couples. In: Boston Lesbian Psychologies Collective eds. *Lesbian Psychologies.* Chicago: University of Illinois Press. Pp. 161–173.

Zak A, McDonald C. 1997. Satisfaction and trust in intimate relationships: Do lesbians and heterosexual women differ? *Psychological Reports* 80(3 Pt 1):904–906.

REPRODUCTIVE HEALTH

Baetens P, Ponjaert-Kristoffersen I, Devroey P, Van Steirteghem AC. 1995. Artificial insemination by donor: An alternative for single women. *Human Reproduction* 10(6):1537–1542.

Brewaeys A, Devroey P, Helmerhorst FM, van Hall EV, Ponjaert I. 1995. Lesbian mothers who conceived after donor insemination: A follow-up study. *Human Reproduction* 10(10):2731–2735.

Chan RW, Raboy B, Patterson CJ. 1998. Psychosocial adjustment among children conceived via donor insemination by lesbian and heterosexual mothers. *Child Development* 69(2):443–457.

Daniels KR, Burn I. 1997. Access to assisted human reproduction services by minority groups. *Australia and New Zealand Journal of Obstetrics and Gynaecology* 37(1):79–85.

Englert Y. 1994. Artificial insemination of single women and lesbian women with donor semen. Artificial insemination with donor semen: Particular requests. *Human Reproduction* 9(11):1969–1971.

Ford C, Clarke K. 1998. Sexually transmitted infections in women who have sex with women. Surveillance data should include this category of women [letter]. *British Medical Journal* 316(7130):556–557.

Gordon S, Snyder CW. 1989. *Personal Issues in Human Sexuality: A Guidebook for Better Sexual Health,* 2nd Edition. Boston, MA: Allyn and Bacon.

Levy EF. 1996. Reproductive issues for lesbians. In: Peterson KJ, ed. *Health Care for Lesbians and Gay Men: Confronting Homophobia and Heterosexism.* New York: Harrington Park Press/Haworth Press. Pp. 49–58.

Ryding EL. 1992. Lesbian women and gynecological examination. *Nordisk Sexologi* 10(2):116–123.

Skinner CJ, Stokes J, Kirlew Y, Kavanagh J, Forster GE. 1996. A case-controlled study of the sexual health needs of lesbians. *Genitourinary Medicine* 72(4):277–280.

Strong C, Schinfeld JS. 1984. The single woman and artificial insemination by donor. *Journal of Reproductive Medicine* 29(5):293–299.

Trevathan WR, Burleson MH, Gregory WL. 1993. No evidence for menstrual synchrony in lesbian couples. *Psychoneuroendocrinology* 18(5–6):425–435.

Wendland CL, Burn F, Hill C. 1996. Donor insemination: A comparison of lesbian couples, heterosexual couples and single women. *Fertility and Sterility* 65(4):764–770.

SEXUAL BEHAVIOR

Conway M, Humphries E. 1994. Bernhard Clinic meeting need in lesbian sexual health care. *Nursing Times* 90(32):40–41.

Eschenbach DA. 1993. Bacterial vaginosis and anaerobes in obstetric–gynecologic infection. *Clinical Infectious Diseases* 16:S282–S287.

Hurlburt D, Apt C. 1993. Female sexuality: A comparative study between women in homosexual and heterosexual relationships. *Journal of Sex and Marital Therapy* 19:315–327.

Kinsey A, Pomeroy WB, Martin CE, Gebhard PH. 1953. *Sexual Behavior in the Human Female.* Philadelphia: W.B. Saunders.

Klein F. 1993. *The Bisexual Option,* 2nd Edition. New York: Harrington Park Press/Haworth Press.

Laumann EO, Gagnon JH, Michael RT, Michaels S. 1994. *The Social Organization of Sexuality: Sexual Practices in the United States.* Chicago: University of Chicago Press.

Leiblum SR, Rosen RC, eds. 1988. *Sexual Desire Disorders.* New York: Guilford Press.

Michaels S. 1996. The prevalence of homosexuality in the United States. In: Cabaj RP, Stein TS, eds. *Textbook of Homosexuality and Mental Health.* Washington, DC: American Psychiatric Press. Pp. 43–63.

Rankow E. 1996. Sexual identity vs. sexual behavior. *American Journal of Public Health* 86(12):1822–1823.

Schreurs Karlein MG. 1993. Sexuality in lesbian couples: The importance of gender. *Annual Review of Sex Research* 4:49–66.

SEXUALLY TRANSMITTED DISEASES

Berger BJ, Kolton S, Zenilman JM, Cummings MC, Feldman J, McCormack WM. 1995. Bacterial vaginosis in lesbians: A sexually transmitted disease. *Clinical Infectious Diseases* 21(6):1402–1405.

Carroll N, Goldstein RS, Lo W, Mayer KH. 1997. Gynecological infections and sexual practices of Massachusetts lesbian and bisexual women. *Journal of the Gay and Lesbian Medical Association* 1(1):15–23.

Edwards A, Thin RN. 1990. Sexually transmitted diseases in lesbians. *International Journal of STD and AIDS* 1:178–181.

Institute of Medicine. 1997. *The Hidden Epidemic: Confronting Sexually Transmitted Diseases.* Washington, DC: National Academy Press.

Kellock D, O'Mahony CP. 1996. Sexually acquired metronidazole-resistant trichomoniasis in a lesbian couple. *Genitourinary Medicine* 72(1):60–61.

Lampon D. 1995. Lesbians and safer sex practices. *Feminism and Psychology* 5(2):170–176.

Marrazzo JM, Stine K, Handsfield HH, Kiviat NB, Koutsky LA. 1996. Epidemiology of sexually transmitted diseases and cervical neoplasia in lesbian and bisexual women. *18th Conference of the National Lesbian and Gay Health Association,* Seattle, WA, July 13–16.

Marrazzo JM, Stine K, Kuypers J, Handsfield HH, Koutsky L. In preparation. Infection with human papillomavirus as determined by a PCR-based method and serology among women who have sex with women.

O'Hanlan KA, Crum CP. 1996. Human papillomavirus-associated cervical intrepithelial neoplasia following lesbian sex. *Obstetrics and Gynecology* 4(P2):702–703.

Robertson P, Schachter J. 1981. Failure to identify venereal disease in a lesbian population. *Sexually Transmitted Diseases* 8(2):75–76.

Russell JM, Azadian BS, Roberts AP, Talboys CA. 1995. Pharyngeal flora in a sexually active population. *International Journal of STD and AIDS* 6(3):211–215.

SUICIDE

Brent DA. 1995. Risk factors for adolescent suicide and suicidal behavior: Mental and substance abuse disorders, family environmental factors, and life stress. *Suicide and Life-Threatening Behavior* 25(Suppl):52–63.

Erwin K. 1993. Interpreting the evidence: Competing paradigms and the emergence of lesbian and gay suicide as a "social fact." *International Journal of Health Services* 23(3):437–453.

Gibson P. 1989. Gay male and lesbian suicide. In: Feinleib MR, ed. *Report of the Secretary's Task Force on Youth Suicide.* DHHS Pub. No. 89-1622. Washington, DC: U.S. Government Printing Office. Pp. 3-110–3-137.

Hammelman TL. 1993. Gay and lesbian youth: Contributing factors to serious attempts or considerations of suicide. *Journal of Gay and Lesbian Psychology* 2:77–89.

Hershberger SL, D'Augelli AR. 1995. The impact of victimization on the mental health and suicidality of lesbian, gay, and bisexual youths. Special Issue: Sexual orientation and human development. *Developmental Psychology* 31(1):65–74.

Hershberger SL, Pilkington NW, D'Augelli AR. 1996. Categorization of lesbian, gay, and bisexual suicide attempters. In: Alexander CJ, ed. *Gay and Lesbian Mental Health: A Sourcebook for Practitioners.* New York: Harrington Park Press/Hayworth Press. Pp. 39–59.

Millard J. 1995. Suicide and suicide attempts in the lesbian and gay community. *Australia and New Zealand Journal of Mental Health Nursing* 4(4):181–189.

Moscicki EK, Muehrer P, Potter LB. 1995. Introduction to supplemental issue: Research issues in suicide and sexual orientation. *Suicide and Life-Threatening Behavior* 25(Suppl):1–3.

Muehrer P. 1995. Suicide and sexual orientation: A critical summary of recent research and directions for future research. *Suicide and Life-Threatening Behavior* 25(Suppl):72–81.

Olson ED, King CA. 1995. Gay and lesbian self-identification: A response to Rotheram-Borus and Fernandez. *Suicide and Life-Threatening Behavior* 25(Suppl):35–39.

Proctor CD, Groze VK. 1994. Risk factors for suicide among gay, lesbian, and bisexual youths. *Social Work* 39(5):504–513.

Remafedi G, French S, Story M, Resnick MD, Blum R. 1998. The relationship between suicide risk and sexual orientation: Results of a population-based study. *American Journal of Public Health* 88(1):57–60.

Rotheram-Borus MJ, Fernandez MI. 1995. Sexual orientation and developmental challenges experienced by gay and lesbian youths. *Suicide and Life-Threatening Behavior* 25(Suppl):26–34.

Ryan C, Futterman D, eds. 1997. *Adolescent Medicine: State of the Art Reviews. Special Issue on Lesbian and Gay Youth: Care and Counseling* (8)2 Philadelphia: Hanley and Belfus, Inc.

Saunders JM, Valente SM. 1987. Suicide risk among gay men and lesbians: A review. *Death Studies* 11:1–23.

Shaffer D, Fisher P, Hicks RH, Parides M, Gould M. 1995. Sexual orientation in adolescents who commit suicide. *Suicide and Life-Threatening Behavior* 25(Suppl):64–71.

Workshop on Suicide and Sexual Orientation. 1995. Recommendations for a research agenda in suicide and sexual orientation. *Suicide and Life-Threatening Behavior* 25(Suppl):82–94.

TRAINING AND EDUCATION

Atkins DL, Townsend MH. 1996. Issues for gay male, lesbian, and bisexual mental health trainees. In: Cabaj RP, Stein TS, eds. *Textbook of Homosexuality and Mental Health.* Washington, DC: American Psychiatric Press. Pp. 645–655.

Bauman KA. 1996. More on gay and lesbian people in our teaching environment [editorial; comment]. *Family Medicine* 28(1):57–58.

Murphy BC. 1991. Educating mental health professionals about gay and lesbian issues. Special Issue: Coming out of the classroom closet: Gay and lesbian students, teachers, and curricula. *Journal of Homosexuality* 22(3–4):229–246.

Murphy BC. 1992. Educating mental health professionals about gay and lesbian issues. *Journal of Homosexuality* 22(3–4):229–246.

Robb N. 1996. Medical schools seek to overcome "invisibility" of gay patients, gay issues in curriculum [see comments]. *Canadian Medical Association Journal* 155(6):765–770.

Robinson G, Cohen M. 1996. Gay, lesbian and bisexual health care issues and medical curricula [editorial; comment] [see comments]. *Canadian Medical Association Journal* 155(6):709–711.

Sanders GL. 1997. Calgary curriculum on gay and lesbian issues [letter]. *Canadian Medical Association Journal* 156(2):166.

Stein TS, Burg BK. 1996. Teaching in mental health training programs about homosexuality, lesbians, gay men, and bisexuals. In: Cabaj RP, Stein TS, eds. *Textbook of Homosexuality and Mental Health*. Washington, DC: American Psychiatric Press. Pp. 621–631.

Telljohann SK, Price JH, Poureslami M, Easton A. 1995. Teaching about sexual orientation by secondary health teachers. *Journal of School Health* 65(1):18–22.

Tesar CM, Rovi SL. 1998. Survey of curriculum on homosexuality/bisexuality in departments of family medicine. *Family Medicine* 30(4):283–287.

Townsend MH. 1997. Gay and lesbian issues in graduate medical education. *North Carolina Medical Journal* 58(2):114–116.

Townsend MH, Wallick MM, Cambre KM. 1991. Support services for homosexual students at U.S. medical schools. *Academic Medicine* 66(6):361–363.

Townsend MH, Wallick MM, Cambre KM. 1996. Follow-up survey of support services for lesbian, gay, and bisexual medical students. *Academic Medicine* 71(9):1012–1014.

Townsend MH, Wallick MM, Pleak RR, Cambre KM. 1997. Gay and lesbian issues in child and adolescent psychiatry training as reported by training directors. *Journal of the American Academy of Child and Adolescent Psychiatry* 36(6):764–768.

Wallick MM, Cambre KM, Townsend MH. 1992. How the topic of homosexuality is taught at U.S. medical schools. *Academic Medicine* 67(9):601–603.

VIOLENCE (INCLUDING DOMESTIC VIOLENCE AND CHILD ABUSE)

Butke M. 1995. Lesbians and sexual child abuse. In: Fontes LA, ed. *Sexual Abuse in Nine North American Cultures: Treatment and Prevention*. Thousand Oaks, CA: Sage Publications. Pp. 236–258.

Cameron P, Cameron K. 1995. Does incest cause homosexuality? *Psychological Reports* 76(2):611–621.

Coleman VE. 1994. Lesbian battering: The relationship between personality and the perpetration of violence. *Violence and Victims* 9(2):139–152.

Garnets L, Herek GM, Levy B. 1990. Violence and victimization of lesbians and gay men: Mental health consequences. Special Issue: Violence against lesbians and gay men: Issues for research, practice, and policy. *Journal of Interpersonal Violence* 5(3):366–383.

Garnets L, Herek GM, Levy B. 1993. Violence and victimization of lesbians and gay men: Mental health consequences. In: Garnets LD, Kimmel DC, eds. *Psychological Perspectives on Lesbian and Gay Male Experiences. Between Men—Between Women: Lesbian and Gay Studies*. New York: Columbia University Press. Pp. 579–597.

Griffith PL, Myers RW, Cusick GM, Tankersley MJ. 1997. MMPI-2 profiles of women differing in sexual abuse history and sexual orientation. *Journal of Clinical Psychology* 53(8):791–800.

Hammond N. 1988. Lesbian victims of relationship violence. Special Issue: Lesbianism: Affirming nontraditional roles. *Women and Therapy* 8(1–2):89–105.

Herek GM. 1991. Stigma, prejudice, and violence against lesbians and gay men. In: Gonsiorek JC, Weinrich JD, eds. *Homosexuality: Research Implications for Public Policy*. Newbury Park, CA: Sage Publications. Pp. 60–80.

Herek GM. 1994. Heterosexism, hate crimes, and the law. In: Costanzo M, Oskamp S, eds. *Violence and the Law. Claremont Symposium on Applied Social Psychology,* Vol. 7. Thousand Oaks, CA: Sage Publications. Pp. 89–112.

Herek GM, Berrill KT, eds. 1992. *Hate Crimes: Confronting Violence Against Lesbians and Gay Men.* Newbury Park, CA: Sage Publications.

Human Rights Campaign. 1998. Fighting Anti-Gay Hate Crimes [WWW Document]. URL http://www.hrc.org/issues/hate/index.html (accessed February 12, 1998).

Klinger RL, Stein TS. 1996. Impact of violence, childhood sexual abuse, and domestic violence and abuse on lesbians, bisexuals, and gay men. In: Cabaj RP, Stein TS, eds. *Textbook of Homosexuality and Mental Health.* Washington, DC: American Psychiatric Press. Pp. 801–818.

Lechner ME, Vogel ME, Garcia-Shelton LM, Leichter JL, Steibel KR. 1993. Self-reported medical problems of adult female survivors of childhood sexual abuse. *Journal of Family Practice* 36(6):633–638.

McCauley J, Kern DE, Kolodner K, Dill L, Schroeder AF, DeChant HK, Ryden J, Derogatis LR, Bass EB. 1997. Clinical characteristics of women with a history of childhood abuse: Unhealed wounds. *Journal of the American Medical Association* 277(17):1362–1368.

Miller BA, Downs WR, Gondoli DM. 1989. Spousal violence among alcoholic women as compared to a random household sample of women. *Journal of Studies on Alcohol* 50:533–540.

Orzek AM. 1988. The lesbian victim of sexual assault: Special considerations for the mental health professional. Special Issue: Lesbianism: Affirming nontraditional roles. *Women and Therapy* 8(1–2):107–117.

Otis MD, Skinner WF. 1996. The prevalence of victimization and its effect on mental well-being among lesbian and gay people. *Journal of Homosexuality* 30(3):93–121.

Pilkington NW, D'Augelli AR. 1995. Vicimization of lesbian, gay, and bisexual youth in community settings. *Journal of Community Psychology* 23(1):34–56.

Renzetti CM. 1992. *Violent Betrayal. Partner Abuse in Lesbian Relationships.* New York: Sage Publications.

Renzetti CM. 1994. Understanding and responding to violence in lesbian relationships. Part III. *Treating Abuse Today* 4(1):20–24.

Renzetti CM. 1996. The poverty of services for battered lesbians. In: Renzetti CM, Miley CH, eds. *Violence in Gay and Lesbian Domestic Partnerships.* New York: Harrington Park Press/Haworth Press. Pp. 61–68.

Stahly GB, Lie GY. 1995. Women and violence: A comparison of lesbian and heterosexual battering relationships. In: Chrisler JC, Hemstreet AH, eds. *Variations on a Theme: Diversity and the Psychology of Women.* Albany, NY: State University of New York Press. Pp. 51–78.

Waldner-Haugrud LK, Gratch LV. 1997. Sexual coercion in gay/lesbian relationships: Descriptives and gender differences. *Violence and Victims* 12(1):87–98.

Waldner-Haugrud LK, Gratch LV, Magruder B. 1997. Victimization and perpetration rates of violence in gay and lesbian relationships: Gender issues explored. *Violence and Victims* 12(2):173–184.

Weingourt R. 1998. A comparison of heterosexual and homosexual long-term sexual relationships. *Archives of Psychiatric Nursing* 12(2):114–118.

Wertheimer DM. 1992. Treatment and service interventions for lesbian and gay male crime victims. In: Herek GM, Berrill KT, eds. *Hate Crimes: Confronting Violence Against Lesbians and Gay Men*. Newbury Park, CA: Sage Publications. Pp. 227–240.

WORK

Dellinger K, Williams CL. 1997. Makeup at work: Negotiating appearance rules in the workplace. *Gender and Society* 11(2):151–177.

Diamant L, ed. 1993. *Homosexual Issues in the Workplace*. Washington, DC: Taylor and Francis.

Morgan KS, Brown LS. 1993. Lesbian career development, work behavior, and vocational counseling. In: Garnets LD, Kimmel DC, eds. *Psychological Perspectives on Lesbian and Gay Male Experience*. New York: Columbia University Press. Pp. 267–286.

Shachar SA, Gilbert LA. 1983. Working lesbians: Role conflicts and coping strategies. *Psychology of Women Quarterly* 7(3):244–256.

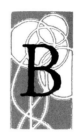

Workshop Agenda

Workshop on Lesbian Health Research Priorities

Georgetown University Conference Center
3800 Reservoir Road, N.W.
Washington, D.C.

October 6–7, 1997

Monday, October 6

9:00 a.m.   **Welcome and Introductions**
Ann Burgess, D.N.Sc., Chair, Committee on Lesbian
Health Research Priorities, University of Pennsylvania

9:30 a.m.   **An Overview of Lesbian Health: Historical and
Developmental Perspectives**
Donna Futterman, M.D., Adolescent AIDS Program,
Montefiore Medical Center, and Deptartment of Pediatrics,
Albert Einstein College of Medicine

10:00 a.m. Lesbians as a Diverse Population: Who Are We Talking About?
Moderator: Judy Bradford, Ph.D.

Lesbians: Defining the Population
Meaghan Kennedy, M.P.H., Centers for Disease
Control and Prevention

Who Is Lesbian? (The Low Interrelationships Among
Sexual Orientation, Sexual Behavior, Years Out,
Disclosure of Sexual Orientation, and Participation in the
Lesbian Community)
Esther Rothblum, Department of Psychology,
University of Vermont

Economic Issues for Lesbians
Lee Badgett, University of Massachusetts and
Institute for Gay and Lesbian Strategic Studies

11:15 a.m. The Contextual Framework: Barriers to Conducting Research on Lesbian Health
Moderator: Bruce McEwen, Ph.D.

Ethical Issues in Conducting Research with Lesbians
Larry Gostin, Georgetown University Law Center

Research on Lesbian Health: Challenges for University
Researchers
Caitlin Ryan, Washington, D.C.

Researcher and Community Collaboration: Issues and
Barriers to Working Together
Joyce Hunter, D.S.W., Community Liaison Program,
HIV Center for Clinical and Behavioral Studies, and
Department of Psychiatry, Columbia University

12:15 p.m. LUNCH

1:00 p.m.   **Designing Studies on Lesbian Health**
Moderator: Larry Norton, M.D.

Designing Effective Studies of Lesbian Health Issues
  Susan Cochran, Ph.D., M.S., Department of
  Epidemiology, University of California, Los Angeles
  School of Public Health

Challenges and Opportunities in Research Design
  Jocelyn White, M.D., Oregon Health Sciences
  University

Health Services Research: Working with Hard-to-Reach
Groups
  Debra Rog, Ph.D., Center for Mental Health Policy,
  Vanderbilt Institute for Public Policy Studies

Research Design and Causation
  Margaret Rosario, Ph.D., Department of Psychology,
  City College, City University of New York

2:30 p.m.   **Scheduled Public Testimony**

Methodological Issues in Research on Lesbian Health
  Alice Dan, Ph.D., Center for Research on Women and
  Gender, University of Illinois at Chicago

Strategies for Obtaining Representative Samples/
Measurement of Sexual Orientation
  Ann Pollinger Haas, Ph.D., Department of Health
  Services, Lehman College, City University of
  New York (representing the Women's Health Survey)

Involving Communities in Research on Lesbian Health
  Amelie Zurn, M.S.W., Silver Spring, Maryland

2:50 p.m.   Cancer and Lesbians
Deborah J. Bowen, Ph.D., Division of Public Health
Sciences, Fred Hutchinson Cancer Research Center

3:20 p.m.   BREAK

3:30 p.m.   Scheduled Public Testimony

Lesbians and Cancer
Beverly Baker, Mautner Project for Lesbians with
Cancer

Lesbian Experiences and Breast Cancer
Linda McGehee, Ph.D., R.N., Georgia State
University School of Nursing

**3:45 p.m.   Sexually Transmitted Diseases—An Issue for
Lesbians?**
Jonathan Zenilman, M.D., Infectious Disease Division,
Johns Hopkins University School of Medicine

**4:15 p.m.   The Challenges of Providing Health and Mental
Health Services to Lesbians: Issues of Access and
Barriers to Care**
Moderator: Gloria Sarto, M.D.

Joan Waitkevicz, M.D., Gay Women's Focus,
Beth Israel Medical Center, New York

Teresa Cuadra, M.D., Gay Women's Focus,
Beth Israel Medical Center, New York

4:45 p.m.   Scheduled Public Testimony

Integrating Sexuality into Health Care and the Need for
Information on Lesbian Health
Christopher Portelli, J.D., Sexuality Information and
Education Council of the United States

Lesbian Health Curriculum for Medical Schools
Devi O'Neill, Center of Excellence for Women's
Health, University of California Medical Center at
San Francisco

Implications for Health Care Service and Delivery and
Lesbians' Access to Care
Beverly Saunders Biddle, M.H.A., National Lesbian and
Gay Health Association

Cultural Proficiency: A Cornerstone to the Success of
Managed Care
Nancy Kennedy, Dr.P.H., Office of Managed Care,
Center for Substance Abuse Prevention, SAMHSA

5:15 p.m.   Final Questions

5:30 p.m.   Adjourn

Tuesday, October 7

9:00 a.m.   Opening and Welcome
Ann Burgess, D.N.Sc., Chair, Committee on Lesbian
Health Research Priorities, University of Pennsylvania

9:15 a.m.   Instrumentation and Disclosure
Moderator: Sam Friedman, Ph.D.

Disclosure of Sexual Orientation in the Nurses' Health
Study II
Patricia Case, Sc.D., Department of Social Medicine,
Harvard Medical School

New Methods for Surveying Sensitive Behaviors
Charles Turner, Ph.D., Research Triangle Institute,
Washington, D.C.

Measuring Health
Ronald Wilson, National Center for Health Statistics
(retired)

10:30 a.m. Mental Health and Substance Abuse Issues for Lesbians
Moderator: Cynthia Gomez, Ph.D.

Overview of Mental Health Issues for Lesbians
Marjorie Sved, M.D., Adult Psychiatry, Dorothea
Dix Hospital, Raleigh, North Carolina

Tonda Hughes, Ph.D., R.N., University of Illinois at
Chicago, College of Nursing
Overview of Substance Abuse Issues for Lesbians

11:15 a.m. HIV/AIDS and Women Who Have Sex with Women
Rebecca Young, National Development and Research
Institute, Inc., and Columbia University Division of
Sociomedical Sciences

11:45 a.m. Scheduled Public Testimony

Lesbians and HIV: The Invisible Crisis
Amber Hollibaugh, Women's Education Services/
Lesbian AIDS Project, Gay Men's Health Crisis

12:00 noon LUNCH

12:45 p.m. Sampling Strategies for Studies on Lesbian Health
Moderator: Donna Brogan, Ph.D.

Probability Sampling for Research on Lesbian Health
Graham Kalton, Ph.D., Westat, Inc., Rockville,
Maryland

Building Relationships: Sampling Methods for Diverse
Communities
  Elizabeth J. Rankow, PA-C, MHS, Consultant,
  Oakland, California

U.S. Census Data: Uses and Limitations for Research on
Lesbian Health
  Martin O'Connell, Ph.D., Fertility and Family
  Structure Branch, U.S. Bureau of the Census

2:00 p.m.   Scheduled Public Testimony and Final Discussion

Elisabeth Gruskin, Kaiser Permanente

Charlotte Patterson, Ph.D., American Psychological
Association

Nina Carroll, Fenway Community Health Center, Boston
Fenway's Research Experience

Winnie Stachelberg, Human Rights Campaign

3:00 p.m.   Adjourn

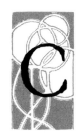

Workshop Participants

Workshop on Lesbian Health Research Priorities

Georgetown University Conference Center

Deborah Aaron, Ph.D.
Department of Epidemiology
University of Pittsburgh

Frances Aranda
Project Coordinator
University of Illinois at Chicago

Lisa Belcher, Ph.D.
Centers for Disease Control and Prevention
Atlanta

Bari Blake
Manager of Outpatient Services
Summit Ridge Hospital
Lawrenceville, GA

Lisa Bowleg, Ph.D.
Senior Research Consultant
Center for Women Policy Studies
Washington, DC

Robin Buhrke, Ph.D.
AAAS Congressional Science Fellow
Duke University
Washington, DC

Nina Carroll
Director of Women's Health
Fenway Community Health Center
Boston

Roberta Cassidy
University of Illinois at Chicago

Jeanine Cogan, Ph.D
Society for the Psychological Study of Social Issues Public Policy Scholar
APA Public Policy Office
Washington, DC

Alice Dan, Ph.D.
Director
Center for Research on Women and Gender
Chicago

Lynda Dattilio, R.N.
Washington, DC

Andrea Densham,
Lesbian Community Cancer Project
Chicago

Kathleen Ethier, Ph.D.
Associate Research Scientist
Yale University

Jack Fitzsimmons, M.D., M.B.A.
Office of Women's Health
Food and Drug Administration
Rockville, MD

Julianna Gonen, Ph.D.
Research Associate
Jacobs Institute of Women's Health
Washington, DC

Elisabeth Gruskin
Kaiser Permanente
Oakland, CA

Ann Pollinger Haas, Ph.D.
Professor
Lehman College
City University of New York

Suzanne Haynes, Ph.D.
Assistant Director for Science
Office on Women's Health
Public Health Service
Washington, DC

Amber Hollibaugh
National Field Director
Women's Education Services
Gay Men's Health Crisis
New York

Rebecca Isaacs
Political Director
National Gay and Lesbian Task Force
Washington, DC

Debbie M. Jackson
Health Policy Analyst
Office of Research on Women's Health
National Institutes of Health
Bethesda, MD

Vivian Jackson
Jackson and Jackson Mental Health and Addiction Consulting
Mitchellville, MD

Wendy Johnson
The Washington *Blade*
Washington, DC

Wanda Jones, Ph.D.
Director
Office of Women's Health
Centers for Disease Control and Prevention
Atlanta

Ellen Kahn, M.S.S.
Director of Lesbian Services
Whitman–Walker Clinic
Washington, DC

Nancy Kennedy, Dr.P.H.
Director, Office of Managed Care
Center for Substance Abuse Prevention
Rockville, MD

Arthur Kennickell
American Statistical Association Committee on Gay and
Lesbian Concerns in Statistics
Washington, DC

Donna Knutson, MSEd, CHES
Section Chief, Division of Cancer Prevention and Control
Centers for Disease Control and Prevention
Atlanta

Howard Kurtzman, Ph.D.
Chief, Cognitive Science Program
National Institute of Mental Health
Rockville, MD

Alysia Kwon
Harvard School of Public Health

Linda McGehee, Ph.D., R.N.
Assistant Professor
Georgia State University School of Nursing

Susan Messina
Freelance Writer–Editor
Washington, DC

Devi O'Neill
Center of Excellence for Women's Health
University of California at San Francisco

Delores Parron, Ph.D.
Associate Director for Special Populations
National Institute of Mental Health
Rockville, MD

Charlotte Patterson, Ph.D.
Department of Psychology
University of Virginia
Charlottesville, VA

Willo Pequegnat, Ph.D.
Associate Director
Office of Research on AIDS
National Institute of Mental Health
Rockville, MD

Vivian Pinn, M.D.
Director
NIH Office of Research on Women's Health
Bethesda, MD

Marj Plumb
Director of Public Policy
Gay and Lesbian Medical Association
San Francisco

Ann Pollinger-Haas, Ph.D
Lesbian Health Fund
Bronx, NY

Christopher J. Portelli, J.D.
Sexuality Information and Education Council of the United States
New York

Bob Roehr
Bay Area Reporter
Washington, DC

Joyce Rudick
Office of Research on Women's Health
National Institutes of Health
Bethesda, MD

Beverly Saunders-Biddle, M.H.A.
Executive Director
National Lesbian and Gay Health Association
Washington, DC

Catherine Simile, Ph.D.
Survey Statistician
National Center for Health Statistics
Hyattsville, MD

Roberta Spalter-Roth, Ph.D.
American Sociological Association
Washington, DC

Tracey St. Pierre
Senior Policy Advocate
Human Rights Campaign
Washington, DC

Winnie Stachelberg
Legislative Director
Human Rights Campaign
Washington, DC

Clint Steib
The Washington *Blade*
Washington, DC

Amelie Zurn, M.S.W.
Mautner Project for Lesbians with Cancer
Silver Spring, MD

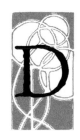

People and Organizations
Submitting Testimony

Deborah Aaron, Ph.D.
Graduate School of Public Health
University of Pittsburgh

Beverly Baker
Mautner Project for Lesbians with Cancer
Washington, DC

Nina Carroll
Director of Women's Health
Fenway Community Health Center
Boston

Alice Dan, Ph.D.
Director
Center for Research on Women and Gender
Chicago

Michelle Danielson
Graduate School of Public Health
University of Pittsburgh

Amber Hollibaugh
National Field Director
Women's Education Services
Gay Men's Health Crisis
New York

Nancy Kennedy, D.P.H.
Director, Office of Managed Care
Center for Substance Abuse Prevention
Rockville, MD

Arthur Kennickell
Committee on Gay and Lesbian Concerns in Statistics
American Statistical Association
Washington, DC

Marguerita Lightfoot
Department of Psychiatry
Division of Social and Community Psychiatry
University of California at Los Angeles

Nina Markovic
Graduate School of Public Health
University of Pittsburgh

Jeanne Marrazzo
University of Washington

Linda McGehee, Ph.D., R.N.
Assistant Professor
Georgia State University School of Nursing

A.D. McNaghten
Stone Mountain, GA

Devi O'Neill
Research Assistant
Center of Excellence for Women's Health
University of California, San Francisco
Northampton, MA

Charlotte Patterson, Ph.D.
American Psychological Association
Washington, DC

Majorie Plumb
Gay and Lesbian Medical Association
San Francisco

Ann Pollinger-Haas, Ph.D.
Lesbian Health Fund
Bronx, NY

Christopher J. Portelli, J.D.
Director of Information
Sexuality Information and Education Council of the United States
New York

Beverly Saunders-Biddle, M.H.A.
Executive Director
National Lesbian and Gay Health Association
Washington, DC

Winnie Stachelberg
Legislative Director
Human Rights Campaign
Washington, DC

Kathleen Stine
Volunteer Medical Director
Sisters Health Services for Sexual Minority Women
Seattle

Amelie Zurn, M.S.W.
Mautner Project for Lesbians with Cancer
Washington, DC

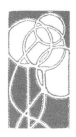

Index

B

Bacterial vaginosis, 73, 102-103
Bisexual women, 4, 22-23, 27, 31, 32
    HIV seroprevalence, 76
    illicit drug use, 82, 83
    reproductive health studies, 106-107
Body mass index (BMI), 57, 64, 67, 68
Breast cancer, 21, 46, 64, 65, 67, 141,
    142
Buddhism, 24, 25
Bureau of Labor Statistics National
    Longitudinal Surveys, 128

C

Cancer, 46, 47, 54. *See also specific forms*
    of cancer
    literature on, 177
    prevention studies, 112-113
    research recommendations, 86
    risk factors, 55, 56, 64-67, 86
Cardiovascular disease, 42, 46, 62, 68,
    86, 112-113
Catholicism/Catholics, 25, 28
Centers for Disease Control and
    Prevention, 1, 14, 18, 140
    lesbian research and programs, 142,
    162-163
    Office of Women's Health, 19
Cervical cancer, 66-67, 70, 73, 142
Chicago Women's Health Study, 102
Childhood sexual abuse, 58-59, 70, 77,
    81
Children and adolescents
    coming-out process, 51-52
    development of sexual identity, 50-51
    heterosexual activity, 78
    literature on, 170-173
    raised in lesbian households, 53-54
    sexuality studies, 149
    suicide, 52, 110-111

Chlamydia, 70, 72-73, 78
Civil rights protection, 39
Clearinghouses on lesbian health, 163
Colon and rectal cancer, 64, 67
Coming out
    age and, 48-49
    coping mechanisms, 51
    cultural contexts of, 24, 49-50, 55
    to family, 24, 49
    fear of, 6, 44-45, 49
    to health care providers, 6, 40, 44-45
    lesbian academics, 138
    process, 48-50, 51-52
Committee on Lesbian Health Research
    Priorities, 17, 18
Conferences on Health Survey Methods,
    162
Confidentiality, 9, 13, 113, 128-129, 150
    n.12, 152-153, 161, 162
Confucianism, 24, 25
Contextual barriers to research, 135-136
    career ramifications, 8, 136-138
    funding to study lesbian health, 8, 9,
    97, 137, 139-140, 153
    mentors for lesbian researchers, 8,
    138-139, 164
    publishing and disseminating findings,
    14-15, 140-144, 153, 161
    strategies for overcoming, 14-15, 144,
    163-164
    training and education of researchers,
    14-15, 163-164, 203-204
Coronary Artery Risk Development in
    Young Adults, 62 n.10
Cultural competency of health care
    providers, 5, 41, 42-44, 157

D

Death, causes of, 46, 47, 68
Definition of lesbian, 21-23
    Committee, 4-5, 17, 25-33

O

Office of Management and Budget, 149
Oral contraceptive use, 56, 57-58, 64, 67, 68
Osteoporosis, 112-113
Ovarian cancer, 64, 67
Overweight and obesity, 56, 57, 62, 64, 65, 68, 102-103

P

Pap tests, 6, 21, 42, 66-67
Partners, lesbian. *See also* Domestic partner benefits
  alcohol use, 81
  legal recognition of, 41
  relationships, 199-200
Pregnancy history, 56, 57, 64, 65
Prejudice and discrimination
  and coming out, 49
  laws against, 37
  lesbian researchers, 136
  prevalence in U.S., 5, 35-37
  research used for, 151
  studies of, 106-107
Prevalence of being lesbian, 23, 26, 28-29, 57
Preventive health care, 45-46, 104-105, 112-113
Professional associations, provider, 44
Prostitution, 78
Protective factors for health, 6, 10, 13-14, 63, 68, 85, 156
Protestants, 28
Providers. *See* Health care providers
Public liaison group, 18

R

Racial discrimination/racism, 61-62

Racial/ethnic minorities
  cancer risk, 64
  coming out, 49-50, 55
  and dimensions of same-sex sexuality, 3-4, 29
  perspectives of sexual orientation, 23-25
  research needs, 13, 117-118, 146, 156, 157, 160-161
  studies of lesbians of, 13, 54-55, 70, 106-109, 129, 180-182
  triple jeopardy, 61, 106-107
Religion. *See also specific religions*
  and dimensions of same-sex sexuality, 28-29
  influences on attitudes, 24, 25
Reproductive health, literature on, 200-201
Research on lesbian health
  adolescents, 153
  barriers, *see* Contextual barriers to research
  community–researcher collaboration, 8, 145-148
  conferences, 14, 162-163
  ethical issues, 150-153
  funding, 7, 11-12, 141, 144, 148-150, 158
  importance, 2-3, 20-21
  informed consent, 153, 162
  longitudinal, 99
  methodologies, *see* Methodological issues in research
  needs and recommendations, 10-11, 50, 81, 84-87, 99, 156-164
  racial and ethnic minorities, 54-55
  uses, concerns about, 151, 162
Risk factors for lesbian health
  beliefs and misconceptions, 2, 21, 63, 65, 72-73, 76-77
  communication with providers and, 43

and HIV/AIDS, 77-78, 102-107,
110-111
and menstrual synchrony in couples,
112-113
and mental health, 102-103
and reproductive health, 106-107
and STDs, 74-75, 102-103
Sexually transmitted diseases (STDs), 54,
66, 67-75, 78, 86, 102-105, 110-
111, 149, 201-202
Smoking, 42, 55-57, 64, 67, 68, 81
Social networks and support systems, 63,
77, 125
Socioeconomic status, 13, 62, 70, 156,
160-161
Sodomy laws, 37, 39
Stanford University, 141
Stigmatization, 5. *See also* Prejudice and
discrimination
of conducting research, 136, 137
of lesbian academics, 137-138
research data used for, 152
and stress, 21
Stress, 3, 21, 59-62, 63, 65, 68, 81
Substance abuse, 54, 77, 79, 86-87. *See
also* Alcohol use; Illicit drug use
Suicide, 51-52, 69-70, 110-111, 202-203
Survey of Family Growth, 117
Syphilis, 70, 72-73

T

Taoism, 24, 25

U

University of North Carolina, 149
University of Washington, 78
University of Wisconsin, 141
U.S. Census of Population and Housing,
128
Uterine cancer, 64

V

Violence against gay men and lesbians,
36, 42, 49, 59, 61, 70, 204-206

W

Whitman Walker Clinic, Washington,
D.C., 142
Women's Health Initiative, 55, 57, 112-
113, 114, 127, 128, 139
Work, literature on, 206
Workshop
agenda, 1-2, 18, 207-213
participants, 18, 215-222
written testimony, sources, 19, 223-
226

Y

Yale University, 142
Young Women's Christian Association,
142
Youth Risk Behavior Study, 160